THE BUZZ ON™

SEX, DATING & RELATIONSHIPS

Rusty Fischer

LF LEBHAR-FRIEDMAN BOOKS
NEW YORK • CHICAGO • LOS ANGELES • LONDON • PARIS • TOKYO

The Buzz On Sex, Dating & Relationships

Lebhar-Friedman Books
425 Park Avenue
New York, NY 10022

Published by Lebhar-Friedman Books
Lebhar-Friedman Books is a company of Lebhar-Friedman, Inc.

Printed in the United States of America

Library of Congress Cataloging-in-Publication Data

      Fischer, Rusty.
      The buzz on sex, dating & relationships / Rusty Fischer.
      p. cm
      Includes index.
      ISBN: 0-86730-815-X (alk. paper)
      1. Dating (Social customs) 2. Dating (Social customs)--Humor. 3. Man-woman relationships.
      4. Man-woman relationships--Humor. I Title: Buzz on sex, dating, and relationships. II. Title.

      HQ801 .F56 2000
      306.73--dc21   00-058360

Produced by Progressive Publishing
Editor: John Craddock; Creative Director: Nancy Lycan; Art Director: Peter Royland
Designers: Angela Connolly, Vivian Torres, Lanette Fitzpatrick

Visit our Web site at lfbooks.com

THE BUZZ ON™

SEX, DATING & RELATIONSHIPS

ACKNOWLEDGMENTS

The author dutifully wishes to thank the following for their contributions to this book:

Patrick Glynn, of Wireless Flash News, whose timely and topical news stories appear courtesy of WIRELESS FLASH, 827 Washington Street, San Diego, California 92103, and can also be found at http://www.flashnews.com.

Chris White, several of whose Top-5 lists appear in this book and who was a countless inspiration for those that don't! Chris is owner of TopFive.com, at http://www.topfive.com.

Haythum Raafat Khalid, who has graciously allowed us to use the quotes found in this book, which also appear on his Web site, Famous Quotations Network: http://www.famous-quotations.com.

Brenda Ross, Web goddess and dating expert extraordinaire, whose list of sample personal ads appear in this book and can also be found at her excellent Web site, Brenda's Dating Advice for Geeks, at http://www.geekcheck.com.

Johnnie Luevanos, Publishing Coordinator at Universal Studios, who graciously allowed us to use the quotes from *Casual Sex*, *Mallrats* and *That Old Feeling*, Copyright © 2000 by Universal City Studios, Inc. Courtesy of Universal Studios Publishing Rights, a Division of Universal Studios Licensing, Inc. All rights reserved.

Thanks to the friendly folks at http://www.women.com for providing illuminating survey results on the ongoing battle of the sexes.

And, finally, a whopping big thanks to "Bootsy," from Bootsy's Sexuality Survey: http://www.geocities.com/SouthBeach/Dunes/7202/poll.html. If it's sexy and it's a survey, Bootsy's got it!

THE BUZZ ON
SEX, DATING & RELATIONSHIPS

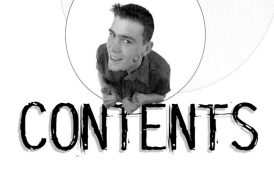

CONTENTS

intro
DATING PREFACE

So, you've finally decided to break down and read The Buzz On Sex, Dating & Relationships. Great. Super. Congrats. Now, quit looking for the dirty pictures and focus. Focus! All right, obviously, you've purchased this book for your "friend," that lovable (albeit "loveless") loser who hasn't had a date in three years, thinks "What's your sign?" is a viable pick-up line, and is seriously considering actively recruiting a mail-order bride . . . or becoming one.

Well, you and your "friend" are in luck. Contained within these lofty pages are the dating basics: flirting, kissing, one-night stands, body language, spicing up your love life, personal ad acronyms, tips for succeeding in your office romance, and even that hottest new trend, cybersex.

Wait, don't go! This isn't another one of those Dummies' or Idiot's guides full of useless lists, voluminous theories, and enough tables, pie charts, and graphs to fill a Microsoft annual report. Sure, we've provided plenty of advice to help you find a date, not to mention enough facts for you to impress your prospective dates with, but we've also given you true-life stories from people just like you: Dateless in Dayton. Clueless in Chicago. Idle in Idaho. Sexless in Scranton. Lonely in Lancaster. Frustrated in Fresno. Crying in Kalamazoo. Numb in New York.

You'll thrill to our collection of Valentine's Date Disasters. Nod your head at our true-life Blind Date Horror Stories. Smile in appreciation of our collection of anecdotes full of enough Lounge Lizards, Hard-drive Hotties, Restless Romeos, and Jilted Juliets to fill a Dating Impaired convention center.

And, just when you think all of this helpful information is getting just a little too helpful, we've thrown in a few tasteless Top-5 lists just to make things a little more interesting.

So, if you're **ready** to romance . . .

If you're **set** to finally become lucky in love . . .

And if you've got a comfortable seat under your lonely butt, let's **go**!

TOP-5 REASONS TO READ THIS BOOK:

5 Now that NBC's cancelled *Freaks & Geeks*, what else is there to do?

4 It's cheaper than a date, and twice as "satisfying."

3 You wasted so much money on all those bad blind dates, they repossessed your TV.

2 Your Mom bought it for you and is standing over your shoulder with a cattle prod.

1 Your membership in the "She Woman Man Hater's Club" has finally expired.

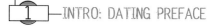

SCREAM 9.5, OR:
EVERYTHING I NEEDED TO KNOW
ABOUT ROMANCE
I LEARNED FROM HORROR MOVIES

What better way to introduce a book on sex, dating, and relationships than with . . . horror! Well, *horror movies*, that is.

Because when you think about it, most hot-blooded American college students learned all they needed to know about relationships from that most respected of all sources—the B-Grade horror movie.

Yes, it's in classics such as *Chopping Mall*, *The Dorm That Dripped Blood*, and *Girl's School Screamers* that students learned safety basics, such as:

• Never walk backward wearing only your bra and panties all alone in the girl's locker room at midnight holding a newspaper whose headline reads: CAMPUS KILLER ON THE LOOSE!

• Never date the captain of the cheerleading squad or the captain of the football team unless, of course, you want to end up like one of the characters in such cinematic classics as *Spikes in the Football Captain's Helmet* and *Cheerleader Cutlets*.

Observant college freshman, therefore, realize that parading around alone late at night and/or dating such ill-fated social pillars (no matter how hot a prospect it may seem when attending your first pep rally) is sure to end in only tragedy, pain, and numerous trips to the cemetery.

> "There's a **monster** in your chest. It's a **really** nasty one. And in a **few** hours, it's gonna **burst** its way through your rib cage, and **you're gonna die**. Any questions?"
>
> —Ripley (Sigourney Weaver) in *Alien Resurrection*

Also, thanks to these socially conscious "scary" movies, campus newcomers come to college knowing other immutable truths: Dating your professor is strictly off limits. For no matter how undeniable the pull of attraction may be to this cultural taboo, cinematically schooled college freshmen know that such relationships are definitely doomed. How many times has the innocent, tank-top-clad co-ed slipped in to see her professor just after office hours,

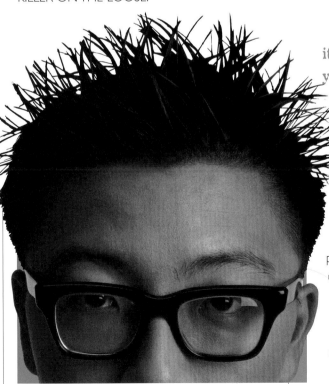

only to find him shedding his skin, revealing the alien life-form beneath, just in time for her to become *his* lab experiment? Isn't *The Professor from Planet Psycho* required viewing for all high school seniors?

Surprisingly, scary movies provide real-life lessons in safe sex as well. Bunk beds, for example, are strictly out of bounds. Any video store-card-carrying college freshman knows that's where horror movie heroes Freddie, Michael, and Jason like to make their "points." Savvy students are also well versed in the plethora of weapons used in the decades-old struggle between would-be freshman fornicators

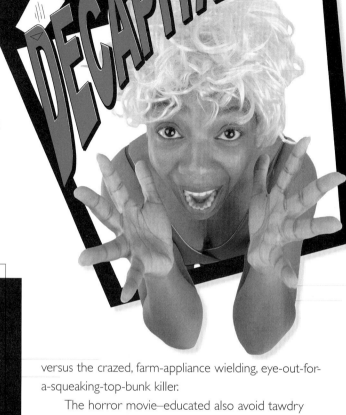

TOP-10 HORROR MOVIES TO AVOID ON YOUR FIRST DATE:

10 **Die! Die! My Darling!**

9 **The Last Horror Film**

8 **Kill, Baby, Kill!**

7 **Theatre of Blood**

6 **Let's Scare Jessica to Death**

5 **Hell Night**

4 **The Devil within Her**

3 **Hatchet for a Honeymoon**

2 **Dressed to Kill**

1 **America's Most Wanted: (Your Date's Name Here)!**

versus the crazed, farm-appliance wielding, eye-out-for-a-squeaking-top-bunk killer.

The horror movie–educated also avoid tawdry trysts in out-of-the-way places. Lover's lanes, dark alleys, and even phone booths are littered with the corpses of college freshmen (usually dashingly portrayed by thirty-year old actors) naïve enough to think that "safe sex" can occur in a world where titles such as *Vending Machine Victims* and *The Broom Closet Killer* scream out: Don't go there!

Aside from obvious dating tips, however, college freshmen learn other, subtler lessons from horror movies. Positive roommate identification, for instance, is one helpful movie hint. Every *Cosmopolitan*-reading co-ed knows not to mix her lipsticks when scrawling on mirrors on a university campus, just as every Joe College knows to check his flip-flops for tarantulas before padding off unsuspectingly to the showers.

And so, while sensitive senators and the Hollywood elite continue their endless debate over violence in movies, the college freshman has just one thing to say to those oft-neglected, B-Grade movie directors: "Keep those chain saws humming!"

"I wish **dating** was like **slaying**. You know, **simple**, direct, **stake** through the **heart**, no **muss**, no **fuss**."

—Xander (Nicholas Brandon) in, *Buffy the Vampire Slayer*

But for those whose "refined" tastes have moved far beyond the B-Grade movie genre and its inherent blood and guts (yeah, right!) there's lots more to learn about the fairer or not so fairer sex. Sure, it's great to know that college professors are a dating no-no and that bunk beds are the romantic equivalent of a buzzing chainsaw, but there's so much more to romance than that.

So, the question begs to be asked: "What do you do now if college romance is just a distant memory?"

Thankfully, *The Buzz On Sex, Dating & Relationships* is a compilation of the latest and greatest information that will help you take that all-important step from Horror Movie 101 to a graduate degree in Dating 2000. So, open the windows, take the garlic off the door, put away your crucifix collection, turn on your favorite lamp, and read on.

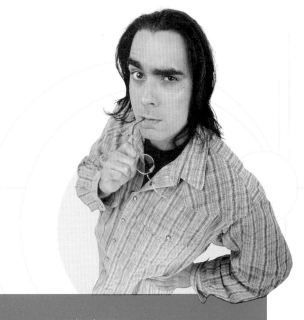

JAWS STILL TAKING BITES OUT OF MOVIEGOER'S SLEEP!

If *Jaws* scared you out of the water or *Psycho* changed your shower habits, a study suggests you probably aren't alone. A survey of one hundred and fifty students at the Universities of Michigan and Wisconsin found that one in four had some lingering "fright" effect from a movie or TV show they saw as a child or a teenager. Some people who saw the thriller about a man-eating shark never went into the ocean again, said Kristen Harrison, a University of Michigan communications professor who co-wrote the study. Ninety percent said they were scared by a TV show or movie from their childhood or adolescence while 26 percent said they still experience "residual anxiety." The younger the children were when they were frightened, it appears, the longer the reaction lasted.

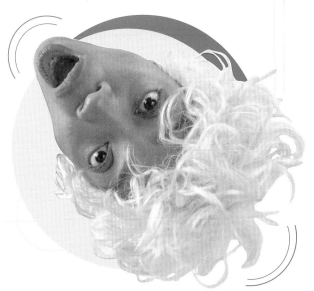

1
ONE
DATING 101

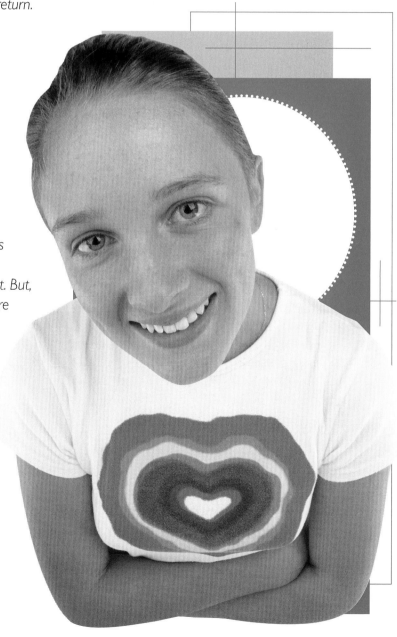

Dating. It used to be so simple, didn't it? When you were just a little thing, a simple stroll up to the local convenience store to buy a cinnamon Jolly Rancher stick for the two of you to share and you could always expect a smile in return.

You could hold hands at the lake or pond or drainage ditch, dangle your feet in the water, and maybe even skinny dip if it was a hot summer night.

In high school, dating was even simpler—school events, parties, socials, dances. They practically made dating mandatory. And if you had a car, look out! Naturally, college was more of the same. Only, minus the adult supervision and plus the hallucinogenics.

But now you're "grown up" and things are different. Sure, you've got the job, the car, the apartment, and the bank account. But, sadly, there are no more keggers. No more pep rallies. No more Jolly Ranchers. It's just you and your wits and your goal: Find Mr. or Miss Right in a sea of Dudley Don'ts and Mindy Mistakes.

Where do you go? How do you tell if he's the one? What flower should you send? And who do you call when your carefully laid plans blow up in your face? Can you learn to master the fine art of flirting? Rediscover the magic of kissing? And discover the world of easy aphrodisiacs at your local video store? Sure you can.

DISASTROUS DATES THROUGHOUT HISTORY
(DON'T WORRY, OUR ANCESTORS COULDNT GET IT RIGHT EITHER)

So, another week gone by, another date gone horribly, terribly wrong? Another weekend evening spent rearranging your sock drawer while *Saturday Night Live* blares in the background and even your cat's meow sounds strangely similar to "loser?" Another Sunday spent seriously considering the morning edition's fresh batch of psychotic personal ads as viable dating alternatives?

So by now you're probably feeling a little ... lonely, huh? A little ... sad? Pathetic? Suicidal? Miserable? Defeated? Depressed? Hopeless? Drained? Worthless?

Well don't fret, you're in good company. Very good company. Throughout history, true love has existed as a fleeting wisp that millions have reached for, yet few have actually realized.

Need proof? Simply amble through the musty pages of your moldy Ancient History textbooks. (You saved all those, right?) Ever heard of a certain tainted twosome that the #1 bestseller of all time likes to refer to as Adam and Eve? Their first date didn't go so hot, now did it?

"Well, Eve, where do you feel like going tonight? Garden of Eden?"

"Yeah. We can grab appetizers on the way in. I hear the apples are in season."

They ended up talking to a snake and the rest, of course, is history.

Or how about Samson and Delilah? Talk about a "bad-hair day." You leave the house the strongest man on Earth and come back with a buzz cut and the strength of Pee Wee Herman. Say what you will about *your* last few bad dates, but most likely you still retained 90 percent of your body strength come Monday morning.

So cheer up. It has been worse.

As time marched slowly on, the Earth's population swelled dramatically and afforded ancient women everywhere plenty of toga-wearing eye candy to choose from. Not that they could do anything about it, of course. After all, these were the pre- "I just got 20 million dollars for starring in *Erin Brockovich*" days.

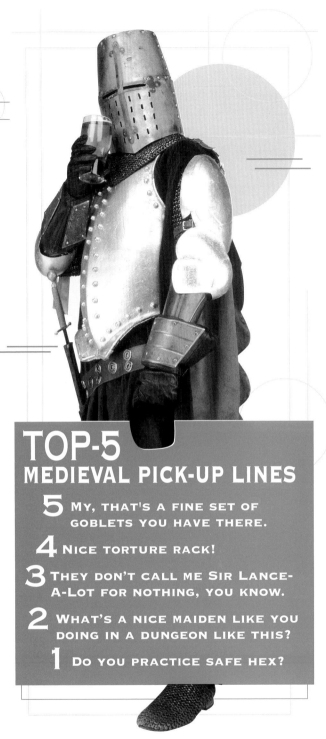

TOP-5
MEDIEVAL PICK-UP LINES

5 MY, THAT'S A FINE SET OF GOBLETS YOU HAVE THERE.

4 NICE TORTURE RACK!

3 THEY DON'T CALL ME SIR LANCE-A-LOT FOR NOTHING, YOU KNOW.

2 WHAT'S A NICE MAIDEN LIKE YOU DOING IN A DUNGEON LIKE THIS?

1 DO YOU PRACTICE SAFE HEX?

Women were considered possessions and even the best of marriages were pure coincidence, since all of them had been arranged long before birth.

Back then, the concept of "dating" was as fantastic a notion as clean underwear (or any underwear, for that matter), toothpaste, double features, and MTV.

Relationships were of a business nature, i.e., "How many oxen dost thou have, Ludicrous Maximus?" And, unless it was with sheep, sex was strictly for procreation and carrying on the family name.

So it was inevitable that as women grew more powerful over time, they were bound to make a few bad choices in their first, few, tentative, hesitant attempts at this new venture known as "dating."

Cleopatra, for example, had a multitude of hard-bodied Egyptian studs to choose from, yet instead she chose to have dalliances with military men. Unfortunately, these power brokers were long on stature but short on life spans.

Joan of Arc, the ultimate "hot date," was yet another historical female who nonetheless pledged her heart to the most eligible bachelor of all. And, before it was all over, she gave new meaning to such future chart-toppers as, "Burning Up" and "Hot Blooded."

Of course, women weren't the only ones making bad decisions back in the "pre-dating" day. Alexander the Great was no doubt the most eligible bachelor of his time and yet his most lasting relationship, according to most sexual scholars, was with his famed horse, Bucephalus! Maybe

that's where Catherine the Great got her notion for ultimate satisfaction.

Despite these brief historical flickers of "girl power" and "alternative lifestyles," however, history continued to march inevitably on with a combination of arranged marriages, loveless partnerships, multiple mistresses, and unrequited passions, not to mention the occasional pillage or plunder.

Along the way, two pesky upstarts thought they'd try their hand at this newfangled "dating" thing. Although both were pretty much jail bait and neither seemed terribly smart, they somehow managed to turn quite a phrase. But Romeo and Juliet were just another in a long series of star-crossed lovers—Tristan and Isolde, Troilus and Cressida, Sid and Nancy. And, had they lived, both would have probably found their combined histrionics and constant sharing of striped tights and hair scrunchies unbearable.

Eventually, however, Columbus (who reportedly had his own share of bad dates) discovered the New World and things really started heating up for all those once-doomed daters. For one thing, interracial dating was the hottest thing going for a while. You didn't really think beads and trinkets were the only things being "exchanged" by those swarthy Spaniards and nubile natives, now did you?

Naturally, such a prime piece of exotic real estate as the New World changed hands countless times and found itself besieged and battled over by countries galore. However, those pesky Puritans who made themselves at home on Plymouth Rock finally and officially settled it for good.

In Colonial times, marriage was strictly encouraged. In fact, bachelors were many times harassed, fined, or even run out of town. Singleness (rhymes with "bliss") was actually seen as the ultimate sign of laziness. After all, the ability to support a wife and family was the single most important event in a young, male colonist's life. Not surprisingly, as it had been throughout history, love was something that developed after the vows, not before, as a natural outgrowth of the commitment to marriage.

During this "passion purgatory" in our nation's history, young people spent nearly a decade choosing a marriage partner. They would meet in church, around the neighborhood, or at home. They grew up together. Young people mingled in mixed-sex groups; young couples could spend time "alone" (if you didn't count the prying eyes of the entire village) walking, riding, or entertaining in the parlor. However, sexual passion was to be contained. Not surprisingly, premarital pregnancy was seen as a sign of weakness and often led to such social stigma as, oh, say, fewer invitations to the local

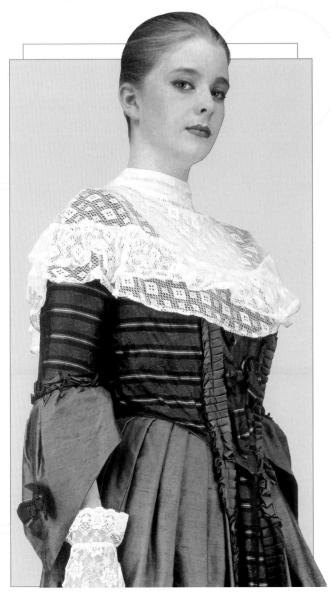

book burning, a scarlet letter or two, and the occasional, unpleasant witch trial.

After the Revolutionary War, America basked in its new-found freedom. Alas, little of this freedom was thrown dating's way. Most of the notable couples from the post-Revolutionary period consist of presidents and their wives: George and Martha, and later Abe and what's her name. During this time, courtship became a way of life and so-called "rules" were imposed on prospective couples. Courtship was strict and often just a formality, as young couples tried energetically to convince themselves that their parents weren't still arranging their marriages. In most cases, courtship involved a lot of boring social engagements at which the boy and the girl were kept occupied from each other until they got to walk home together, supervised, of course, and there was occasionally a little hand holding after a certain amount of time.

Chaperones were prevalent during this era, as were corsets and, as a result, many medical cases of what were thought to be "genital demons," actually were later found to be blue balls. Surprisingly, however, one remnant of this colonial period still remains today: the front porch shuffle. As young couples made it home, cool chaperones often turned their heads so that the young "lovers" could at least grab a quick smooch on the front porch before turning in for the night.

So, perhaps that whole, "Should I kiss her/is she ready, should I/I don't think so, she might be ready/but what if I'm wrong/she'll think I'm a jerk/but if I don't, she'll think I'm gay" routine we all spend so much time worrying about at the end of the night is actually genetic. But then, that's a whole chapter unto itself.

Most likely, since chaperones were unpaid (not to mention frustrating) positions, the practice slowly faded away throughout the end of the 19th Century and the beginning of the 20th. Indeed, by 1920, the centerpiece of American courtship in America was in place—dating. It was informal, unchaperoned, hormone-driven, knicker-nibbling, male-to-female (in most cases) interaction with no specific commitment. (Yippee!)

Not surprisingly, Americans had two monumental developments in modern technology to thank for this sexy situation: the car and the motion picture. Cars represented freedom, and a portable spot to "get busy." Movies, while slightly more public, were also often darker and a much cheaper option for teenagers who had neither the money to buy nor the license to drive a car.

In this respect, little has changed on the modern American dating scene. Kids still neck in cars, people still make-out at the movies. Back in the fifties some genius combined the two and created the drive-in movie theater. Was that guy smart or what?

Accordingly, the 20th Century saw a veritable explosion of famous couples: Scott and Zelda Fitzgerald wrote and drank themselves into literary history (and a few insane asylums). Fred Astaire and Ginger Rogers danced across movie screens to the delight of millions of satisfied ticket-holders—when they could unlock lips long enough to look up at the screen, that is. Elizabeth Taylor and Richard Burton acted, drank, cheated, fought, acted, cheated, drank, acted, cheated, and fought their way through numerous movies, not to mention marriages. Humphrey Bogart and Lauren Bacall were an item on and off-screen. Lucille Ball and Desi Arnaz had, among other things, a hit TV show, little Ricky, and about a zillion fights. And who could ever forget Sonny and Cher? And Gregg Allman and Cher? And Cher and the Bagel Boy?

As times changed, the couples changed as well. The tight-lipped Victorianism of the early 1900s gave way to the flappers and fenders of the Jazz Age. Prohibition may have stopped business at the liquor stores, but the gin joints and blind pigs thrived and so did dating.

Along the way, dating became less of a means to an end (i.e. marriage, remember that?) and more of a means unto itself. The stigma surrounding divorce was slowly eroded by the sheer numbers occurring each year and what was once scandalous (bare feet, then bare knees, then bare thighs, then bare midriffs, then bare backs) slowly became passé. Courtship gave way to cruising, cruising gave way to parking, and parking gave way to "watching the submarine races." Which, of course, in *Happy Days*-speak, was just another "wink, wink, nudge, nudge" term for parking.

Goofy slang was not all that *Happy Days* gave us, however. It also gave us the Fonz. Who, despite being short, goofy, a little slow, and not particularly handsome, quickly became the first *real* TV stud. Sure, that guy from *Hawaii 5-0* and Michael Landon were pretty cool, but a whole generation of girls grew up swooning over the Fonz and, when he almost got serious with Pinky Tuscadero, hearts across the nation braced for disaster. Another favorite couple from TV that really had it going on, and occasionally still do, are Kermit the Frog and Miss Piggy. Sure, they're from two different branches of the animal tree and not particularly compatible, but, like all couples, their off and on again romance is at least realistic.

Of course, like all good things, love in TV Land had to end sometime. Fonzie jumped the shark pit, Pinky never really recovered after that Malachi crunch, and Jim Henson's estate recently sold The Muppets to Germany—*that* should be fun.

And so, as the millennium dawns, new famous couples crop up (and break up) as quickly as a bad case of genital herpes. Hmmm. Coincidence? There's Demi and Bruce. Demi and Brad. Brad and Gwyneth. Gwyneth and Ben. Ben and Matt. Who knows who will be left standing in the end?

There now, doesn't that make you feel a little better?

It doesn't? Well, here's one more boost for your battered emotional ego: just remember how many Hollywood hotties Warren Beatty "had" to go through to find his Mrs. Right. To name just a few, the pre–Annette Bening Warren Beatty has been romantically linked with, among others: Isabelle Adjani, Brigitte Bardot, Candice Bergen, Jacqueline Bouvier-Kennedy-Onassis, Judy Carne, Cher, Julie Christie, Joan Collins, Britt Ekland, Jane Fonda, Melanie Griffith, Goldie Hawn, Bianca Jagger, Diane Keaton, Vivien Leigh, Madonna, Michelle Phillips, Diana Ross, Diane Sawyer, Stephanie Seymour, Carly Simon, Barbra Streisand, Liv Ullmann, Mamie Van Doren, and Natalie Wood. (And we all know the only reason he's never dated Shirley MacLaine is because she's his sister!)

Of course, guys aren't the only ones breaking hearts left and right. After all, at least Warren Beatty only *dated* his stable full of women. But Elizabeth Taylor

went and did him one better: she married each of her misters. To the tune of eight times! Count 'em for yourself: married twice to actor Richard Burton, her other husbands were hotelier Nick Hilton, actor Michael Wilding, filmmaker Mike Todd, singer Eddie Fisher, U.S. Sen. John Warner, and construction worker Larry Fortensky!

Wow, I guess that *doesn't* make you feel any better, now does it? Never mind.

Ladies, how long did it take you to fall in love with your most recent boyfriend/girlfriend?

15 minutes	15%
30 minutes	2%
2 hours	2%
1 day	6%
4 days	5%
1 week	7%
2 weeks	10%
1 month	32%
3 months	21%

Guys, how long did it take you to fall in love with your most recent boyfriend/girlfriend?

15 minutes	22%
2 hours	9%
1 day	9%
4 days	4%
1 week	17%
2 weeks	9%
1 month	9%
3 months	21%

FLIRTING WITH DISASTER

EYE CONTACT

Ah, to be a successful flirt. To bat those dreamy eyes, flex those bulging biceps, and "walk the walk." To have an inexhaustible repertoire of pick-up lines on which to call in any given situation to "close the deal," to "score!"

But what exactly is this thing we call flirting? Basically, it's a polite, perky, sassy way to refer to all that flurry we so love to (secretly) watch on the Discovery Channel at 3 a.m.: the feather-shaking, quirky dancing, neck-biting, circling, whooping, hollering, spitting, fur-flying courtship maneuvering engaged in by our four-legged friends, and otherwise known as "mating rituals."

Naturally, as humans, we've improved on such animalistic adaptations over time. And, as our posture and cranial capacity improved, so did our pick-up techniques. We discovered gold with which to plate massive medallions and thus cover our still-hairy chests or cleavage. We then invented buttons and polyester, only to unbutton them quickly and thus display even more gold and chest hair or cleavage.

We built bars, in which to display our gold, polyester, and chest hair or cleavage. We concocted drinks to "help" seduce each other, songs to set the mood, and aphrodisiacs in case all else fails.

But there is much, much more to flirting than a musky scent and a little muscle-or-rump rippling.

Flirting begins with the eyes. Plain and simple. It doesn't matter if you're wearing thick bifocals or baby-blue colored contacts: the eyes still have "it." Naturally, there is a difference between the necessary act of "making eye contact" and that pesky habit of "staring."

The first means a slow, deliberate gaze from across a crowded room. The second is a blatant attempt to mentally unscrew the subject's eyeballs from their skull sockets and creep inside their cranium for a little close-up soul searching. Of course, if it's your first day in prison, by all means, try the latter. But if you're looking to get lucky (with anyone except Marilyn Manson, that is) in all instances, go for the first.

Eye contact is best made while walking up to somebody (slowly, remember, baby steps) or talking to them (quietly, no shouting).

FURTIVE FLIRTING

DO YOU FLIRT?
YES	68%
NO	32%

IF SO, WHY?
I'M INNOCENTLY FLEXING MY "MUSCLES"	68%
I WANT SOMEONE NEW TO WOO ME OUT OF A TROUBLED RELATIONSHIP	17%
I'M LOOKING FOR TROUBLE	15%

[SURVEY RESULTS COURTESY OF *Women.com*]

Holding the other person's gaze will then communicate the indisputable fact that you are intensely interested in him or her. Again, there's a fine line here between charming and creepy. Both members of the opposite sex enjoy a nice, long exchange of mutual eye contact. It's a sign of respect and admiration. Just remember to blink! And, if you start feeling that your staring contest is going on a little too long, it probably is.

GREAT WHITES

Just below the eyes, once you're finished making pleasant, focused eye contact for eight minutes, is a little thing we humans like to refer to as the mouth. Use it. (No, no, not yet. Quit slobbering all over her. Kissing comes later.) Smile. Grin. Show off those "great whites" of yours. Nothing says "friendly," "together," and "confident" like a nice big smile. Like yawns, smiles are contagious. Even if you're chatting up a sultry, smoky, somber sex siren who has done nothing but glower at her glowing cigarette all evening, smile away. Eventually, unless she's one of those human statue model chicks and she isn't allowed to, she'll catch on.

Of course, listening and smiling go hand in hand. There's no bigger turn-off than an inappropriate smile at the worst possible moment. For instance, if the hunk in black across from you has been talking about his grandmother's funeral for the last half hour, smiling the whole time might make you appear somewhat less than sympathetic, which is never a great flirting tactic.

PICK-UP LINES

Of course, eye contact and smiling are both examples of nonverbal communication, which occasionally serve you well in noisy bars or crowded dance halls. Eventually, however, the crowd will die down and the band will take a break. What then? Well, this is where

those useful little "pick-up lines" you've heard so much about come in handy. Don't worry, they've gotten better over time and, like all things, have improved with age. Over the past eight million years or so, "Ooga booga" gave way to "Oogus boogus," which progressed to "Wanna get together and begat something?" which gave way to "Is that the plague, or are you just gushy all over?"

Hey, you've got to start somewhere. And, despite their bad reputation, pick-up lines are a great ice breaker. Naturally, such lines are intended to open doors, not get them slammed shut in your face. Accordingly, the slow and steady win the race. Unless you're a super stud or heavenly hottie who has the "partner patter" down pat by now (in which case, what are

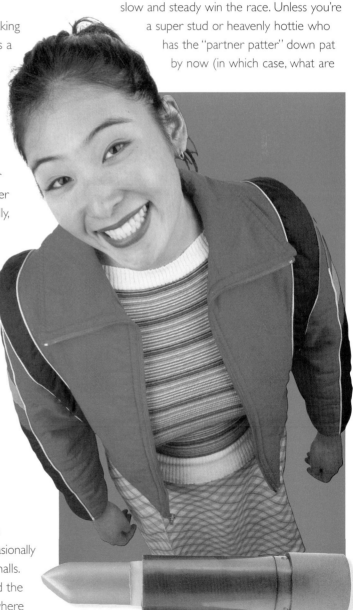

TOP-10 WORST PICK-UP LINES

10 "Are you into casual sex or should I dress up?"

9 "Do you work for UPS, because I just saw you checking out my package."

8 "How do you like your eggs? Poached, scrambled, or fertilized?"

7 "May I end this sentence with a proposition?"

6 "I lost my bed, can I borrow yours?"

5 "Do you believe in love at first sight or should I walk by again?"

4 "Just call me milk, I'll do your body good."

3 "Are you an alien because you are 'out of this world'?"

2 "Hi, I just lost my phone number. Can I have yours?"

1 "I may not be Fred Flintstone, but I bet I can make your bed rock."

you doing here?) your best bet is something simple, like:

"Hi." (Hey, haven't you ever heard of "less is more?")

"Hey, I'm _____, what's your name?" (Nice.)

"Do you want to dance?" (It helps if you're at a wedding or other dance-potential soirée. This might not work at the local library.)

Naturally, smug or flippant lines are often a turn-off unless you precede them with something like, "You're not going to believe this, but I just heard this total loser say . . ." one or more of the following:

"You remind me of a man I used to date." (Quick comeback: "Really, maybe you should go look him up then.")

"Bet I can outdrink you." (Actually, most guys react favorably to this one.)

"I play the field, and I think I just hit a home run with you." (Home run? Doubtful. Strike out? Yes.)

"Your place or mine?" (Try neither, nerd.)

"Can I buy you lunch?" (Check your watch before trying this one.)

Just remember that a pick-up line should fit its speaker. If you're comfortable cracking a joke, go ahead. If not, it might fall flat. And don't try memorizing a big, long speech either. A few words, yes. More than that, you're likely to forget half of it and fill in the missing parts with inappropriate, i.e. sexual, ramblings.

The best pick-up lines are spontaneous. Maybe you're hanging at the local sports bar with your girlfriends, and he's still wearing his jersey from the afternoon softball game when you say something ridiculous like, "Bet a guy like you doesn't strike out too often."

Or maybe it's the post-wedding bash, and she's obviously wearing a gaudy, uncomfortable bridesmaid dress when you casually mention, "I've got a great polyester suit back home that would look super next to that."

On second thought, it's hard to go wrong with a quick "Hi."

FOCUS!

Intensity. This is key to flirtation fruition. The person you are flirting with is the most important person in the world. Period. Without a doubt. (At least, for the minute you are together.) Never mistake flirting for casual conversation anymore than you confuse watered down drinks for a straight shot. Every word counts, but, more important, so do both ears.

Listen. Pay attention. Listen. Watch. Listen. Nod. Listen.

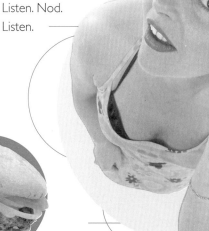

Sympathize. Did we mention, listen? There's nothing sexier than feeling like someone is really listening to what you have to say, especially in today's modern, fast-paced world of selfish conversation and self-promoting memos, e-mails, and phone messages.

Most people assume flirting is all about what they have to say. But maybe they'd be more successful flirts if they paid more attention to what their partner was saying. Try it, you just might like it. If not, hey, hopefully you've got a nice, cool drink to keep you occupied while that bore across from you rambles on and on.

SCAMMING THE DIGITS

Naturally, the goal of flirting is to make further contact. In the past, this was a phone number, i. e. digits. (What did you think we were suggesting, taking home a spare thumb?) Today, of course, phone *numbers* might be a more appropriate term. There are home numbers, work numbers, pager numbers, and cell phone numbers. Of course, the choice is up to you. For safety reasons, most people avoid giving out their home numbers to every Tom, Slick, or Carrie. Work numbers are nice, especially if you have a secretary to screen your calls in case you wake up the next morning with a hangover. Pager numbers are good too, as they can be easily ignored and the un-returned calls blamed on bad batteries.

Today, however, new digits include those perky little e-mail addresses. Many modern singles prefer this new development in the evolution of dating. They pro-vide the least amount of confronta-tion with the most

amount of delete-ability. They're also a great way to practice your partnership patter before you meet again.

Great. Fine. Super. But how do you *get* the digits? Sorry, partner. Unless your other half of the flirting fraction just hands them over after the first drink, there's no easy way out except to just ask. After all, all the person can say is no.

To avoid that, however, try to time your request with the end of your seduction session. Firm is good, forceful isn't. "Gimme your number" isn't really the greatest way to go, unless you say it with a cute, endearing, puppy dog smile and put a question mark at the end. It's probably better to say something like, "Wow, is it last call already? I can't believe it! It's been really nice talking to you. Is there any way I can get your phone number or e-mail address so we can keep in touch?"

If your conquest says "no," well, better luck next time. If you're handed a business card, cheer up. You're halfway there.

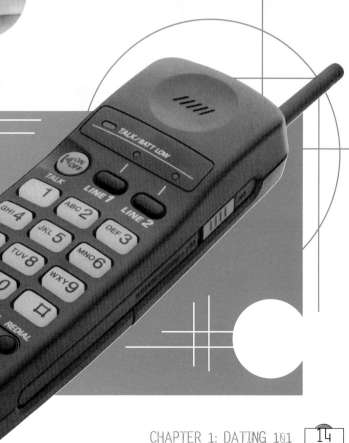

CLOSING THE DEAL

Flirting, after all, is a means to an end. To some, that end is a one-night stand full of hot monkey love and broken furniture. To others, it's merely an enjoyable evening spent in the company of an interesting member of the opposite sex. Either way, how you end your flirtation is entirely up to you. If you feel comfortable prolonging the evening in various stages of undress, so be it. If you prefer a peck on the cheek and a half-hearted, "I'll call you," be our guest. Either way, try to make sure there's some kind of closure at the end of the night, or you're likely to become obsessed with "the one who got away."

Keeping your cool is usually the best way to go here. If you've bored the poor girl out of her skull all night long with basketball statistics and your lackluster curriculum vitae, don't grab her arm when she turns to leave. Thank her for listening and look for somebody a little more desperate. If he falls asleep during the thrilling tales of your glory days as a high school band member, don't douse him with your half-empty margarita. Just put a cocktail napkin (conveniently littered with your e-mail address, phone number, and measurements) under his elbow to make him more comfortable.

Of course, if you've been a successful flirt, your "flirtee" will more than likely be wide-eyed and alert. In which case, congratulations. Your "I'm a Flirt!" certificate is available at the door.

"It is not enough to conquer; one must learn to seduce."

– Voltaire

PUCKER-UP
THE LOST ART OF KISSING

Just like snowflakes, no two kisses are ever alike. Why, even on the same day, between the same loving couple, kisses can be as different as black and white. Just check out their "good morning," pre-coffee peck on the cheek and compare it with their night cap after a steamy evening full of oysters and *Cinemax After Dark* suck-face session!

Still, the simple philosophy behind a kiss is always the same: I love you! Sure, there are different kinds of kisses: The devout person's pucker planted on the Pope's ring. The maternal kisses of a mother on her child's fuzzy

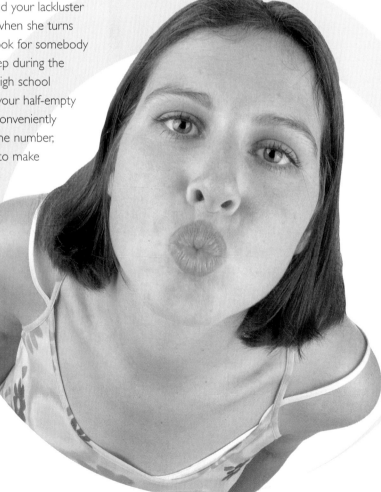

head. The friendly kiss of two people who are meeting for lunch. And, while some kisses may be more casual than others, the love is still there, lurking just behind those pearly whites.

Sadly, many of us have lapsed into a kind of "kissing comfort zone," where our lips have gotten lazy and our tongues are rarely used. For most of us, after all, there are only three kinds of kisses: The "See You After Work" kiss in the morning. The "Honey, I'm Home" kiss in the evening. And, finally, the "I'm in the Mood" kiss on Saturday night.

Naturally, it's only this last kiss that anyone really puts any time and effort into. But let's not forget, kissing has been around since Adam and Eve. And there's a lot more to it than just a pucker or a smack.

DAILY VARIETY

Whoever said, "variety is the spice of life" was obviously talking about kissing. Sure, we've all got the same equipment: two lips to pucker up, two rows of teeth to nibble with, a tongue for probing purposes, and a nose that always seems to zig when it should have zagged. But what about the rest of our bodies? Have we forgotten about eyelashes, ears, necks, limbs, stomachs, chests, and more?

After all, only one half of a pucker partnership needs to use their lips. The target can be anywhere on the recipient's body. Sure, it might be a little forward of you to start slobbering over your blind date's toes before you've even made it to the restaurant. But why not try kissing her hand at the end of the night instead of rushing all the way to third base? Originality is the key. Project the unexpected.

Ladies, why wait on the guy to pucker up? Many is the man who'd fall head over heels for the gal with enough chutzpah to kiss *his* hand out of the blue. Of course, try and make sure he's washed it first. You know how guys are.

TIMING IS EVERYTHING

Kisses, like everything else, have a time and a place. For instance, funerals aren't a great time for kissing. Hospitals aren't a great place. The first is a strictly "hugs only" event, the second is for those snazzy doctor's masks. Likewise, first dates are rarely a great time for a real kiss. Unless, of course, it's been one heck of a first date.

And even if it has been a great first date, isn't patience still a virtue? If there's meant to be a second date, then a good hug or a peck on the cheek before you walk in your door is a pleasant way of hinting at more to come. If the date was doomed from the start, why set yourself up for a 99.9 percent chance of rejection by making that awkward stretch toward a quickly turning head? However, plenty of other places are ripe for the opportunity of a well-timed kiss.

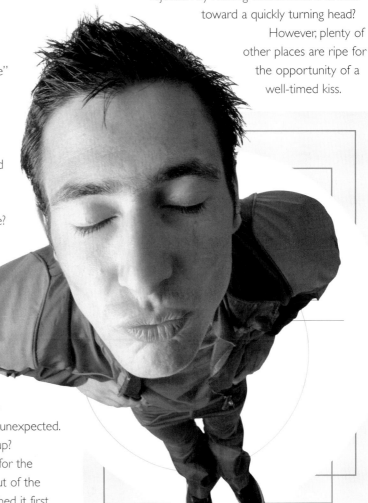

TAKE ME OUT
TO THE BALLGAME

Obviously, there's a big kissing difference between watching a sporting event on TV and seeing it unfold in person. Despite your preference for hockey over basketball, or football over soccer, live sporting events are fraught with enough emotion to make kissing as pleasant a side effect as that foot-long red-hot or catching a foul ball.

Picture the scenario: it's the bottom of the ninth. Bases are loaded. Your team is down by three runs and a solid grand slam would bring it all home.

Now watch as Casey steps up to bat. Here's the pitch, and the swing. Strike one! Another pitch, another swing. Strike two! Pressure's mounting, your boyfriend's mangling his battered ball cap in his shaking hands as pitch three sails toward the plate and, and, and —crack! Up it goes, higher and higher, the ball sailing for deep center and, and, and —it's over the fence! Home run for the home team.

Now, do you politely sit down and fan yourself with the program? Heck no! You shout. You yell. You scream. Your boyfriend embraces you in a moment of raw emotion and before you know it the stands are empty and your lips are chapped from the greatest kiss of your life!

Tennis, anyone?

MISTLETOE
MADNESS

Holidays are another great time for kissing. Naturally, Valentine's Day dates, no matter how abominable, are often capped off with the obligatory kiss between two embattled losers who are just so thankful that the evening is over

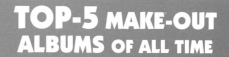
they'd kiss a frog. New Year's Eve is another big kissing holiday. 4, 3, 2, 1! Start smooching! However, the duration is sadly lacking. Not to mention, the law of supply and demand at many New Year's Eve parties makes for some interesting pucker partners: boy, girl, boy, boy, girl, girl. You get the picture.

However, for the most kissing potential in the least amount of time, there's nothing better than the mistletoe madness that sweeps America during the holiday season. Those little sprigs of white-balled greenery crop up everywhere it seems. From grocery stores to pharmacies, from night clubs to restaurants.

Got a crush on that hottie in accounting? Get a mutual friend to steer her under the mistletoe at the office Christmas party and let the sparks (or slaps across the face) fly. Either way, you're sure to get a jolt!

Can't wait that long? Why not make everywhere you go a mistletoe stop? Sure, why not? Nowadays, those sensual sprigs are sold everywhere from convenience stores to florists, from gas stations to bookstores.

Place a sprig in your purse and pull it out over that hunk on the subway. Have some ready in your jacket pocket and whip it out when it comes time to pay that cute little cashier at your daily lunch counter.

Hey, the mistletoe might be plastic, but your lips aren't.

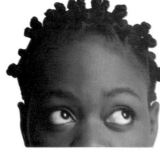

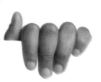

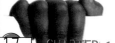

FORGET ABOUT THE BRIDE
KISS EVERYONE!

Is there any setting more ripe for a pleasant pucker than a wedding? All of those flowers. The champagne. The band (good or bad). The champagne. The ceremony. The tissues. The champagne.

Weddings are an emotional time for everyone involved. Fathers giving away daughters. Mothers giving away sons. Groomsmen sucking courage out of flasks hidden in their tuxedos. Bridesmaids shaking from nicotine withdrawal. Guests who have skipped breakfast trying to quiet the rumbles in their stomachs and checking their watches. Needless to say, the reception is a great place to unwind, relax, and—kiss.

Like a bubble, a wedding reception is an insular world unto itself. Time stands still as the band plays on and the drinks flow. Men weep openly and hug enthusiastically. Women cry freely and hug even more enthusiastically. And, as time marches on, the cake gets cut, the bride and groom head off to their lives together, and men stop hugging other men and women take over. And vice versa, of course. First it's relatives, then it's friends, and soon it's tall, dark, and handsome strangers under the cake table.

Hey, who ever said yawning was the only thing you could do with your mouth that was contagious?

Surprise SURPRISE!

Of course, barring holidays, weddings, and sporting events, kissing is an equal opportunity event! Every day can be a kissing day, whether it's a stolen peck after church on Sunday or a silent smooch in a darkened theater.

Need some more ideas for places to smack that surprise kiss? Try these:

— After whipping his butt in racquetball.
— In the Romance aisle at the local video store.

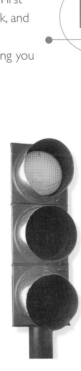

— Can you say "red light?" Damn, there's another one! We've hit every one so far.
— While taking that weekly Saturday morning stroll through the park.
— Standing in line at Burger King.

After all, kissing is free. And there's no waiting around for two weeks after you special-order the equipment. It's all right there, under your nose. Literally.

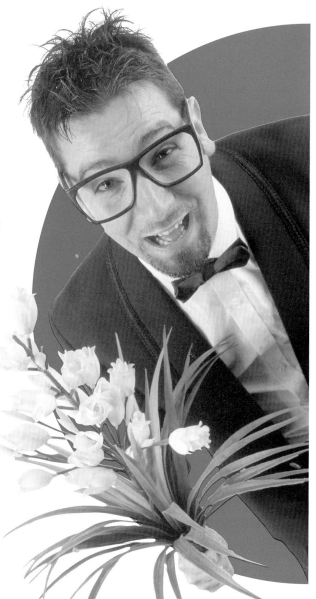

DAISY DICTIONARY: FLOWERS
AND THEIR MEANINGS

Today's overflowing arsenal of dating ammunition is varied and plentiful. Thanks to the Internet, we've got electronic greeting cards, do-it-yourself e-mail love poems, and personal Web pages to declare our undying love like so many miniature billboards dotting the information freeway of love.

Of course, there's always the old standbys, classics such as jewelry, bottles of wine, and the emergency gift, chocolate.

Fine. Great. Super. But when you're ready to stop shooting blanks and start bringing out the "big guns," think flowers. Poppies. Daisies. Pansies. Lilacs. Roses. These are the nuclear warheads in your love arsenal. So what are you saving them for?

The first known written account of the secret, hidden language of flowers can be traced all the way back to ancient Constantinople in the 1600s. The romantic Lady Mary Wortley Montagu, who had spent time in Turkey with her husband, brought

FLOWER POWER

Naturally, some floral facts are as unreliable as they are undeniable. For instance, while the popular carnation has many "real" definitions, the one it most easily conjures up is, "I just ripped this off some guy's tuxedo!" Then again, some flowers actually say what they mean and mean what they say. Feeling crabby? Deliver a mound of fresh crabgrass. Your girlfriend casting a spell on you? Send her some witch hazel. Feeling spicy? How about a cluster of scallions.

Of course, there'll be no mistaking the "frustrating" message you send her along with that fresh bouquet of Texas blue bells!

it back to England in 1716. This language of flowers was translated to French, and *Le Langage des Fleurs* was printed with over 800 floral facts. Of course, the French spiced it up and the English translation at the time of Queen Victoria was censored because it was considered risqué.

A ROSE BY ANY OTHER NAME

Okay, roses are easy. Easy to buy. Easy to send. Easy to interpret. For instance, we all know that the red rose stands for "love." We even know that the yellow rose stands for "friendship." (Haven't we all gotten our share of those before?) Depending on your source, the famed white rose stands for either "fear" or "chastity." Either way, it's nothing you want to see the FTD guy bringing to your door! And, of course, the pink rose stands for "indecision."

"Flowers are words which even a baby can understand."

- Arthur C. Coxe

TOP-5 HIDDEN MEANINGS FOR FLOWER/PLANT GIFTS

5 Mint = your breath needs a car wash.

4 Poison ivy = no sex until that nasty rash clears up.

3 Venus fly trap = that wart on your pinky really bothers me.

2 A dozen red roses = at ten cents each, they'll last as long as the relationship.

1 Sunflower (seeds) = stopped by a convenience store on the way over.

But why stick to a single color? After all, if you can mix the last two bottles of booze in your liquor cabinet (it doesn't matter if it's vodka and scotch), why can't you combine your flowers just as easily? Why be so obvious? Send her a mixed message (is there any other kind?) by combining a red rose surrounded with a few yellow ones. This says one of two things. Either, "I really love being friends with you," or "I'd love to be more than friends with you." Come to think of it, it could also say, "I'm in love with your best friend." But you get the picture.

And women should join the fun too. Flowers weren't only meant *for* you. Send your newest date a few "mixed messages" of your

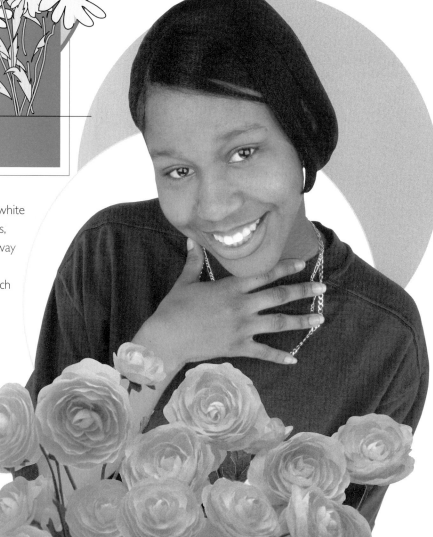

How often does your mate **send** you flowers?

Once a year, usually on Valentine's Day or my birthday **44%**

What are flowers, as in never? **38%**

Once a month, I can clock the florist's delivery after a spat **11%**

Every week on the way home from work **7%**

"faithfulness" just before you head out for that big business trip to Vegas. Then send him a blue violet. Don't want her to forget you while you're at the yearly shareholder's meeting? Send her some forget-me-nots to make that message loud and clear.

Feeling childish (i.e. you're in the mood to dress up like a Catholic schoolgirl to his stern headmaster)? Try a buttercup. Feeling ashamed after your latest beer blowout? Then it's time for a bouquet of peonies. Got a headache even though it's date night? Send him a white poppy and let him know you'd rather "sleep" than sleep together.

own any day of the week. How about a white rose and a yellow rose together? This says, "I'm afraid your chastity is getting in the way of a beautiful friendship."

Hey, who knew you could so say so much with so little?

DON'T OVERLOOK THE OBVIOUS

Looking for something a little more original than roses to send your sweetheart? Good idea. A wider variety of flowers naturally increases the amount of hidden meanings you can convey. Maybe you'd like to express your

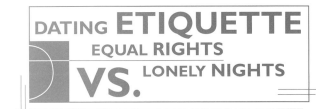

DATING ETIQUETTE
EQUAL RIGHTS
VS. LONELY NIGHTS

KEISHA'S STORY

Keisha Sinclair was tired of hailing her own taxicabs. Or, if her date did have a car, tired of hearing his tires squeal on the pavement outside her apartment building long before he'd even seen if she'd gotten inside safely. She was tired of flagging down waiters in restaurants and, more often than not, paying the tab for dinner and a movie. But mostly, Keisha was just plain tired.

Almost thirty, she'd been on at least five times that many dates in the last few years and the number of men who'd turned out to be gentlemen was running at a paltry .0099 percent. She guessed she was spoiled. Her father had been a gentleman, her mother a lady. She'd simply assumed that the world outside her parents' front door would not be some alternate universe.

Keisha often blamed herself. She was strong, solid, successful, spoke her mind, and favored tasteful dresses and simple jewelry at work and colorful, yet conservative, jeans and silk blouses for play. Maybe guys were scared to pull out her chair, open her car door, or get up off of their lazy behinds when she walked into a room. Maybe they thought they'd offend her.

To help her next date out, she sat down at her glowing laptop one frustrated evening after another disastrous date spent picking out the wine and paying for a taxi 'cause the guy didn't feel like driving ten minutes out of his way. There, frustrated and tired, she wrote down ten items that she considered to be the long lost art of dating etiquette:

1.) Pick up your date — on time!

2.) Pick the restaurant before she gets in the car.

3.) Open her damn door!

4.) Turn off that hip-hop and let a lady listen to some Luther Vandross for a change.

5.) Open her car door when you get there, and the restaurant door on your way inside.

6.) Pull out her chair, unless the joint has a maitre d', and then stand there patiently while he does it.

7.) Ask what she'd like to drink, then order it.

8.) Ask what she'd like to eat, then order it.

9.) Stand up when she leaves, or returns to, the table. Oh, and chew with your mouth closed, use your napkin, and don't smoke until she's done eating.

10.) Pay for dinner, or, at least, go Dutch. Drive her home, and, if she doesn't ask you up for a little Courvoisier and Barry White afterward, at least wait until she gets to her front door before peeling out!

Keisha realized that she could have made it the "100 Tips Of Dating Etiquette," but she was tired and, anyway, she knew most guys' attention spans weren't anywhere near that long! Instead, she wrapped it up at an even ten, e-mailed the list to her computer at work and went to sleep.

The next morning at work, Keisha slyly forwarded her list to a friend's computer. From there, she cut and pasted it into a message from yet another friend's computer, and finally, from there, e-mailed it to her date for the next weekend. Like some cyberspy, she wanted to be careful to cover herself with an electronic trail that couldn't be traced back to her. . . just in case.

Then she waited for Saturday night, and hoped her date had been cramming all week long! It turned out he had.

He showed up at her door (no honking the horn for her as he slowed down to a "gentlemanly" 5 m.p.h.).

And, although he was a full two minutes early, he politely waited until 7 p.m. to knock. He commented on her outfit, handed her a single rose, and gently crooked her arm in his for the walk down the driveway. He opened her door and actually waited until her feet were inside before shutting, not slamming, it. True, there was no Luther playing inside, but he had the jazz station tuned in low, and he didn't smell like a smoker. In fact, from the heady scent of strawberry wafting her way, she judged the cardboard air freshener dangling from his rearview mirror was brand new. She couldn't help but feel flattered.

At the restaurant there was another flurry of door openings, seat pulling, and menu ordering, all done by him, and she wondered why she hadn't thought of her little covert e-mail much earlier.

After dinner, as she instinctively reached for her wallet, he gently covered her hand and guided it back into her purse. As he pulled out his credit card, a business card fell to the floor and, as a return gesture for the most polite date she'd ever been on, she stooped quickly to pick it up before he could. Noticing the shiny computer and technical sounding name on the front, she handed it back with a smile, glad to see that it wasn't for some escort service or topless bar.

"Thanks," he smiled. "I've been having a little trouble with my computer this week and I thought these guys could help. They're supposed to be the best in town."

"Oh, really," she said casually as she toyed with her rich dessert. "What kinds of problems?"

"Oh," he assured her as he left a generous tip, something she hadn't even included in her list. "Nothing serious, I just haven't been able to get my e-mail all week."

Keisha sputtered, "All week?"

"Yeah," he said. "It crashed last weekend and it took me all week to find somebody reasonable. I can only imagine how many messages are piled up. Why? You haven't tried to e-mail me recently, have you?"

But Keisha was speechless. She was too busy trying to remember if there was any Courvoisier in her apartment or not.

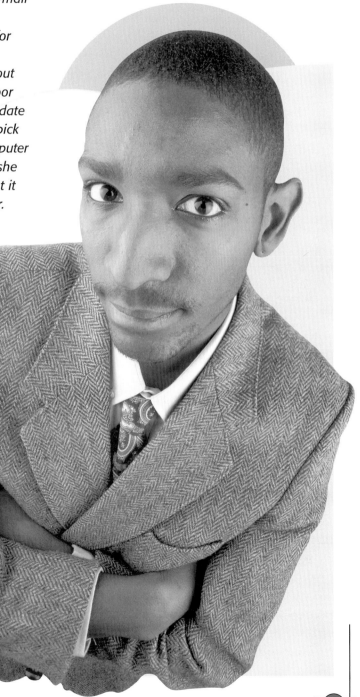

CHAPTER 1: DATING 101 — 24

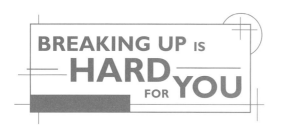

BREAKING UP IS HARD FOR YOU

It's over. Come on, you both know it. Things haven't been right for days, weeks, maybe even months. He's stopped signing your little notes with all those cute little Xs and Os you used to hate. You've stopped sleeping in his oversize T-shirts because you're already trying to sort through what's his and what's yours in the closet. (Just in case you need a quick getaway.) The very sound of his voice raises your hackles. And what about his overabundant toenail clippings on every available surface?

Still, neither of you can say the actual words: "It's over." Is it fear? Comfort? Weakness? Despair? Who knows? Either way, the time has finally come to say, "good-bye." But who first? When? Where?

Okay, so now you're sharing your favorite booth at the little pizza parlor down the street and fighting over the last slice of large veggie pizza while he gently divides the last dregs of a pitcher of beer between your two, frosty mugs.

You sip. You chew. And still, silence reigns. Is he thinking what you're thinking? Mainly, that even though you desperately want to be rid of him, you're scared of what awaits you out there. The bad dates, the blind dates, the *no* dates during that inevitable dry spell.

Is he, like you, dreading your reemergence onto the dreaded dating scene? Is he thinking of all the leeches out there that will be relentlessly hitting on you as soon as they hear you're available? Or, even worse, the very real possibility that nobody hits on you at all? Is he already envisioning the long nights alone spent over a cup of chamomile tea and bad late-night TV?

No, he probably isn't. For one thing, he hates tea. And besides, it's easier for guys. Naturally, he will go through the inevitable string of rebound redheads, busty brunettes, and "brilliant" blondes as he bounces from bar to bar after a long day of the 9 to 5 grind in search of that "comfort zone" he just left behind in you.

No, he'll do fine. It's *you* you're worried about.

Still, it has to be said. Has to be done. And, once you've said it, out loud, without actually crying, he pretends to be crushed and, perhaps for the first time in months, rushes to sit next to you on your side of the scarred booth. There are hugs, maybe a few tears and, what the hell, a fresh pitcher of beer and maybe a sausage calzone to go.

What's it gonna hurt, anyway? After all, you're young, you're wild and, finally, you're free.

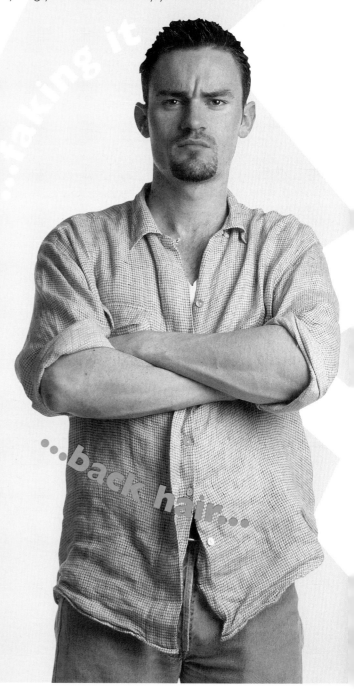

...faking it

...back hair...

Yet still he lingers near your side, tipping that pitcher a few more times as you reminisce together, promising to call, promising to stay in touch even as you leave your favorite downtown restaurant in separate cars.

Perhaps, full of pizza and beer foam and empty of guilt and commitment, your car stereos will play a little louder than usual on the way home. He'll crank up that retro, acid grunge crap you never liked, and you can finally jam to your collection of pseudo folk singer chick CDs as you drive toward bright, single futures.

Alone, but not quite lonely . . . and heading into the great unknown.

To help you forge ahead through that great unknown, we've come up with a "separation sampler" of tips to help you make the transition from happy couple to sane singles a little more smoothly. (No, that doesn't include sending him one of those dead buffalo heart bouquets you heard about on TV the other night, either!)

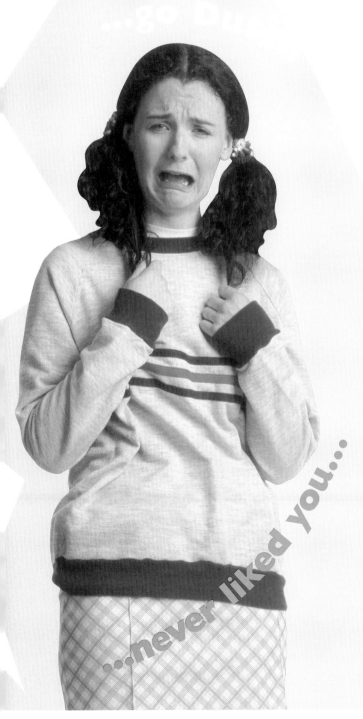

...go Dutch...

...never liked you...

STICKS AND STONES

Naturally, words are as important a part of breaking up as, say, burning his prized baseball card collection or drinking your fifteenth toast to her miserable memory. Sure, you've already said the hardest words: "I can't stand you anymore." (Or something similarly sensitive.) But there's much more to be said if you plan on remaining friends or at the very least speaking to each other ever again.

For instance, it's best not to dwell on your ex's faults. After all, you don't have to put up with them anymore, so why keep harping on them? What do you care if she still snores? You won't be around to hear it. And who cares if he still refuses to change his underwear more than twice a week? You're not hanging around to reap the "benefits" anymore.

Therefore, avoid any critical comments that tend to sound like sour grapes. Even if your ex is spreading rumors all over town, try to rise above his childish behavior and be the polite one. In general, here are a few key phrases to avoid after a break-up:
— "I never liked you anyway."
— "You fool, I was always faking it."
— "You know, if I'd collected all the back hair you left in my bathroom, I could weave a wig by now."
— "My new girlfriend *loves* to go Dutch!"

You get the picture. Anything that sounds a little too "catty" most likely is. And it's never a great idea to burn your bridges. Who knows, you could get a wedding invitation in the mail tomorrow and need a pity date ASAP. And even though your ex-boyfriend's a total heel, he'd sure look good in a tux.

FIVE **BEST** PLACES TO **BREAK UP**

5 At a sold-out rock concert.

4 In front of his parents.

3 Outside of your A. A. meeting.

2 Just before stepping into a cab (that's already pulling away).

1 While he's being awarded First Place at the local pig-calling contest.

ACTIONS SPEAK LOUDER THAN WORDS

As we've just seen, words are an integral part of the entire breaking up process. However, the trick is to not say one thing and then turn around and do another. As in proclaiming passionately, "Of course not, Laura. I'm not ready to sleep with anyone so soon," even as your new girlfriend awaits you giggling and breathless in the bedroom surrounded by an open copy of the *Kama Sutra* and the "Pleasure Dome" kit from the local adult bookstore.

Chances are your close circle of friends will report any and all dalliances posthaste to the offended party, which naturally only lends insult to injury and makes you look like an even bigger jerk than before. Therefore, if you simply must have a passionate one-night stand with that hunky bartender at the nightclub down the street, do it at his place so your roommate doesn't run and tell your ex and break his heart all over again. (Hey, it's the least you can do, considering he's your ex's best friend and all.)

DIVIDE AND CONQUER

The complicated thing about breaking up is that you're not just severing ties with your ex, but your old group of friends as well. Sure, everybody says they'll support you, but just try calling them at the last minute on some Saturday night. Chances are they're already long gone and taking your ex up on his offer to treat them all to front-row seats at the Bruce Springsteen concert.

Naturally, those three or four cozy couples you used to spend your time with won't feel comfortable choosing one of you over the other. After all, it used to be so fun hanging out at the bars, theaters, or clubs as a four-some, six-some, or eight-some. Somehow, three-somes, five-somes, and seven-somes just don't compete. Therefore, the dreaded post-dating division must inevitably occur.

The question remains: "Who gets to keep the friends?" Invariably, the answer is, "Whoever behaves the best." After all, concert tickets and impromptu floral deliveries are one thing, but sitting around your old

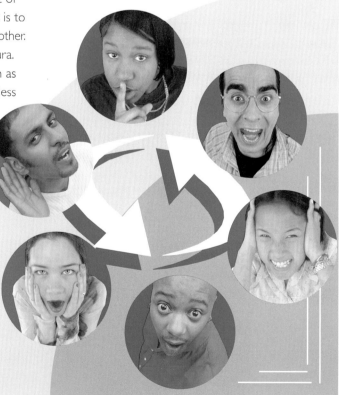

haunts dredging up bad memories and calling your ex every name in the book is not going to endear you to your old friends anymore than showing up with a new lover to take the place of the old. In this case, slow and steady truly wins the race. Remain friends, keep up your routines, and most of all, expect to stay in the loop. Let your ex rant and rave, call names and defame, and chances are, he'll just end up doing it by himself.

TIMING IS KEY

Fine, you've found the right words to say and even the correct actions to go along with them. You've kept the friends or found new ones. Now all that's left is to retrieve that size XL Foo Fighters T-shirt she used to love to sleep in or that Miles Davis CD he liked so much. After all, fair is fair. Just remember that timing is everything. You don't need to rush over to her house the day after you've dumped her and break in through the fire escape just so she won't set fire to that tie you left over there for six months. Likewise, no matter what you think of him twenty-four hours after telling him he never once managed to satisfy you in two years, he's still not giving away the collection of earrings and extra thong underwear you kept in his bottom drawer.

The general rule is to give each other one full week to let things cool down. A seven day week, not a business week. At this point, a polite phone call is in order. (Not a prank call. We said polite!) Something like, "Hi, Bill. How ya been? Great. Super. Listen, I've got a few minutes after work, I was thinking of stopping by and just picking up that suitcase full of toiletries I kept underneath your bed. Would that be all right?"

Chances are, unless the suitcase actually contains priceless coins (or porn) your ex-boyfriend will be glad to get rid of it. If not, give him another week to forget that you dumped him for your old roommate from college and then give him another ring. If he's still stalling, write the darn thing off and run down to the corner drugstore already. If he's that upset, chances are he's already replaced your shampoo with Neet and your toothpaste with Preparation-H anyway!

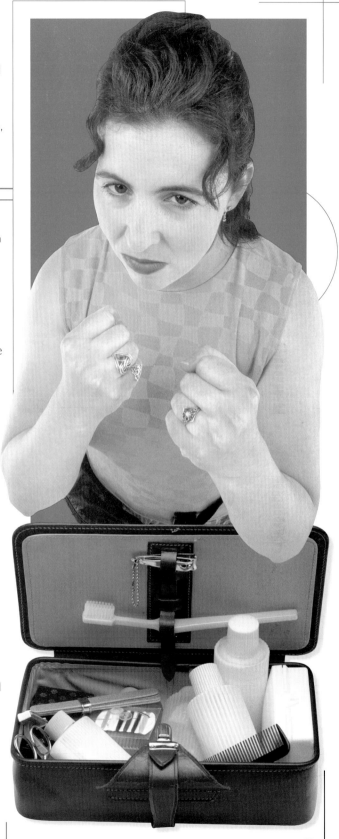

HOLIDATING, OR MERRY EX-MAS!

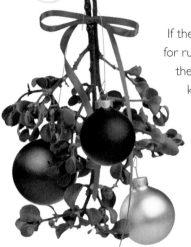

If there's a worse time for running into an ex than the holidays, we'd like to know about it! The remembrances of past gifts, the warm moments shared under the mistletoe, and even the smells associated with the holidays, and each other, are often more than you can bear.

After all, you've broken up, packed it in, moved out, and, more important, moved on. You've split up the friends, given back all of his boxer shorts, and even retrieved that missing jade earring from under his bed. (You've even quit prank calling him at 3 a.m. every morning!) Your tears have all dried up, and you've even lost a few pounds just for spite.

Months have gone by, maybe even years, and still, everything's just hunky dory. But what happens when you run into him again? At the mall? During the holidays?

Or even worse, what happens when all of that "packing it in" and "moving on" results in a brand new boyfriend and, strolling through the mistletoe-bedecked mall, you not only run into your ex for the first time in months, but it's just after he's run into *his* ex? Read on to find out:

TOP-10 HOLIDAY CDs GUARANTEED TO CAUSE A HOLIDAY BREAK-UP (TRUST US!)

10 Jingle Cats
Meowy Christmas

9 The Brady Bunch
Christmas With The Brady Bunch

8 Various Artists
Touched By An Angel: The Christmas Album

7 Ren & Stimpy
Crock O' Christmas

6 Alvin & the Chipmunks
Greatest Christmas Hits

5 Veggie Tales
A Very Veggie Christmas

4 'N Sync
Home For Christmas

3 Barry Manilow
Because It's Christmas

2 John Tesh
A Romantic Christmas

1 Kathie Lee Gifford
Rock 'N' Tots Café Christmas

MERRY
EX-MAS

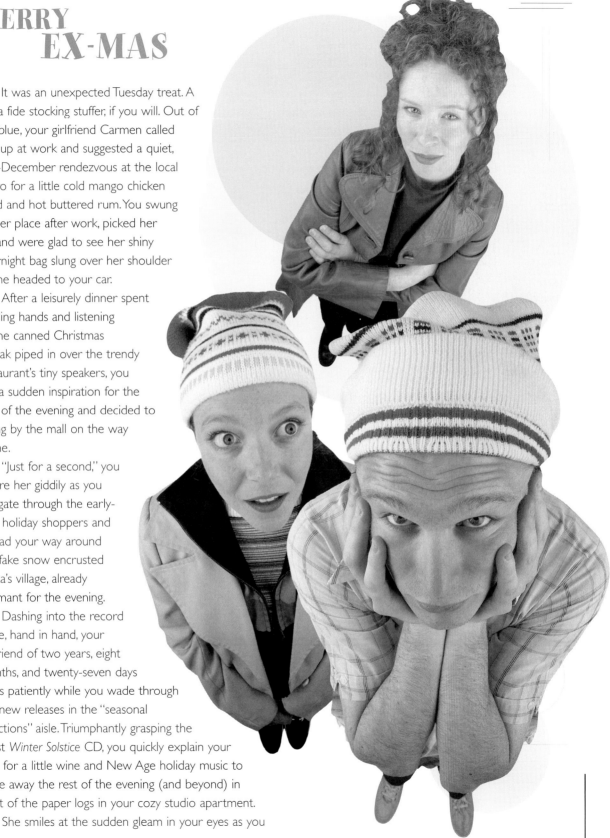

It was an unexpected Tuesday treat. A bona fide stocking stuffer, if you will. Out of the blue, your girlfriend Carmen called you up at work and suggested a quiet, mid-December rendezvous at the local bistro for a little cold mango chicken salad and hot buttered rum. You swung by her place after work, picked her up, and were glad to see her shiny overnight bag slung over her shoulder as she headed to your car.

After a leisurely dinner spent holding hands and listening to the canned Christmas Muzak piped in over the trendy restaurant's tiny speakers, you got a sudden inspiration for the rest of the evening and decided to swing by the mall on the way home.

"Just for a second," you assure her giddily as you navigate through the early-bird holiday shoppers and thread your way around the fake snow encrusted Santa's village, already dormant for the evening.

Dashing into the record store, hand in hand, your girlfriend of two years, eight months, and twenty-seven days waits patiently while you wade through the new releases in the "seasonal selections" aisle. Triumphantly grasping the latest *Winter Solstice* CD, you quickly explain your plan for a little wine and New Age holiday music to while away the rest of the evening (and beyond) in front of the paper logs in your cozy studio apartment.

She smiles at the sudden gleam in your eyes as you

present your overpriced music selection to the oversized, frizzy-haired cashier, who promptly recognizes you and screams, loud enough for the mall's fake Santa to hear all the way from home, "Max? Compton? Is that really you? Why, I haven't seen you since you gave me that nasty case of crabs and dumped me for that cheerleader six Valentine's Days ago!"

As your girlfriend wrenches her hand out of yours with a sickening thud you try and reconcile the middle-age mass in front of you with the long limbed hottie who'd broken your heart nearly seven years ago by announcing that you'd given her crabs. When, after all, you didn't even know what crabs were and actually thought she was referring to a lovely date you'd once spent together at Red Lobster!

Later, not even refraining from scratching their flaring crotches in front of you, your ex-friends explained quite sensitively that she'd been sleeping around with several of them for months and that they'd never told you because, in their words, "We thought you knew." The cheerleader, of course, was just a rebound relationship and ended shortly thereafter.

You try explaining all of this to your girlfriend as you race to catch up with her after signing your credit card slip and tossing it at the ex-crab-ridden, ex-hottie. In fact, she has just started actually listening to you when a dashing figure who'd obviously just graduated from male model school calls out her name from across the food court and thus impedes your breathless explanation.

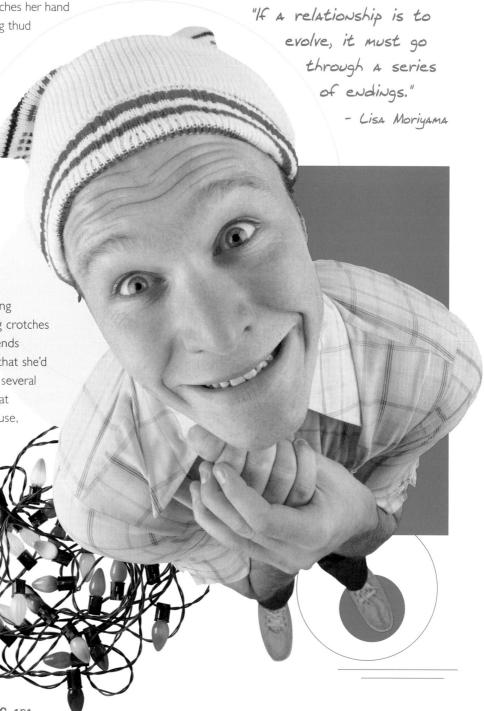

"If a relationship is to evolve, it must go through a series of endings."
— Lisa Moriyama

While the three of you stand just outside of the deserted Santa's village, the two of them reminisce steamily about their once passionate affair several years ago. And, far from breaking up with her over crabs, genital warts, or any other appalling STDs, your girlfriend actually broke up with him. And it's quite apparent, to you anyway, that he's never gotten over it.

From the looks of it, neither has she!

When she finally does get around to introducing you, as her "friend," no less, the lanky pretty boy in his trendy clothes and stylish sunglasses stares down at your premature bald spot and smirks knowingly, indicating the many ways in which he is obviously superior to you.

The two ex-lovers exchange business cards (not to mention smoldering glances) as he dashes off to get his Rolex cleaned in the mall jewelry shop, but not before making plans to "do lunch" with your girlfriend. (With the emphasis, clearly, on the word "do." Bastard!)

The ride back to your place is colder than the December air outside your icicle light balcony and just as frigid. When you turn around after pouring the wine to find the extra pillow and flannel comforter folded neatly on the couch, you realize suddenly that your romantic plans for the evening are further out of reach than the North Pole.

As you drift off to a fitful sleep, staring at the blinking Christmas tree lights and wondering how such a wonderful holiday evening could go so terribly, horribly wrong, you realize dreamily that you never even got to listen to that new *Winter Solstice* CD.

TOP-10 GREATEST HOLIDAY MAKEOUT CDs

10 Bing Crosby
White Christmas

9 Ella Fitzgerald
Ella Fitzgerald's Christmas

8 Boney James
Boney's Funky Christmas

7 Boyz II Men
Christmas Interpretations

6 Aaron Neville
Soulful Christmas

5 Mel Torme
Christmas Songs

4 Lou Rawls
Christmas Is The Time

3 Lena Horne
Christmas

2 Luther Vandross
This Is Christmas

1 Elvis Presley
Blue Christmas

2
GETTING PERSONAL

You can't have a relationship without getting personal. Well, you can, but we're not going there.

Intimacy is a great thing, but first you have to meet someone (usually). There are many ways to meet the man or woman of your dreams, but personal ads can be a good place to start. Over the last few years, the "personals" have gone from being the place where the lunatic fringe lurked to an accepted way to sort through an intriguing string of dating possibilities.

Of course, personal ads aren't for everybody. In general, the inherent risk element involved in meeting and greeting a total stranger who only knows you through your clever turn of phrase (not to mention your knack for putting a positive spin on the fact that you're missing a few teeth and your left leg doesn't quite reach the floor) tends to attract the "hale and hearty" types. Is that you?

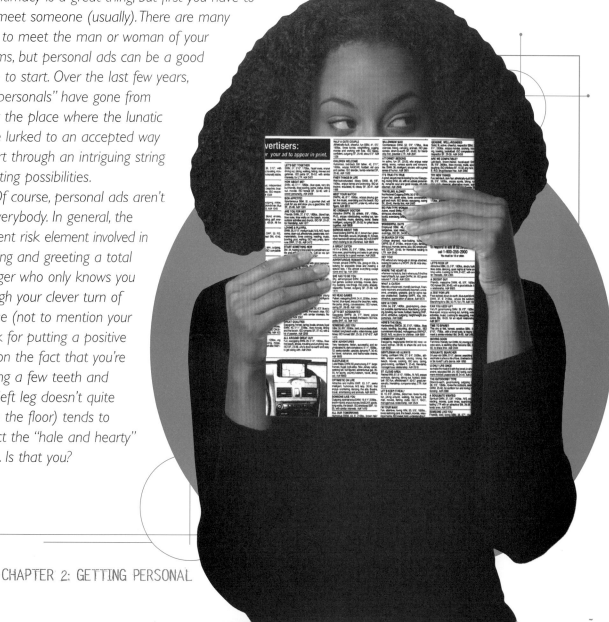

PERSONALLY SEEKING:

So, you've decided to write a personal ad. Whoops, sorry, that's just the deafening sound of everyone around you laughing out loud. Okay, now where were we? Right, the ad. Well, you're obviously past the point of rational thought so, right about now, you could probably use a little help.

"Lead us not into temptation. Just tell us where it is; we'll find it."

— Sam Levenson

Of course, we can do our best to help you write your very own personal ad. However, regardless of whether you plan to place it in the local paper, the back of *Rolling Stone,* or on the Internet, please take our advice: before you do please, please, *please* give the bar scene one more shot. You never know, that female impersonator you met last week might just be looking good right about now.

TITILLATING TITLES

Okay, this is the first thing people will read. So make it good. But not *too* good. After all, you don't want to get so many responses that you don't have time to answer them all. (What if Brad Pitt was the very last person to write and you'd already stopped halfway down the list with Arnold Schlemelmacher from Hoboken?)

In general, avoid cliche phrases like "Looking for Mrs. Wrong," "Sick of the Singles Scene," "Tired of Being Lonely, Desperate, Sad, Scared, Stupid, and Afraid," etc. On the other hand, don't get too witty. You don't want to come off as Shakespeare and then have to keep up *that* charade for the rest of your life.

Think of your personal ad title as one of those movie trailers. You know, "In space, no one can hear you scream." Something that catches the readers' attention and makes them want to keep reading. For help, take a look at other ads and see what titles catch your eye. And, remember: stay clear of negative titles, like "Hey. Come on. Why is no one writing to me? Huh? Come on, guys . . . guys?"

Even if no one is writing to you, no one ever will if you start off sounding like such a total, sorry-assed, sad sack at the get-go.

TOP-5 PERSONAL ADS THROUGHOUT HISTORY:

5.) "Religious zealot seeks shameless sinner to break 11th commandment. Meet me behind the burning bush."

4.) "Sun Goddess seeks same to make Sun God jealous."

3.) "Aquaman seeks Swamp Thing for watersports. I've got the flippers, you bring the snorkel!"

2.) "SWM whose wife was just turned into pillar of salt seeks someone less spicy!"

1.) "Military leader seeks same for threesome. Bring horse!"

SOBERING STATISTICS

As you've probably already noticed (after all, they're what most people read first), the majority of personal ads contain statistics such as your age, height, marital status, weight, whether you smoke or drink, number of sexually transmitted diseases, etc.

There are two schools of thought concerning personal ad statistics. If you're looking for a quick "meet and greet" in which you plan to rely on your silver tongue to wine, dine, and bed your innocent "victim," by all means, stack the deck. Lie, cheat, fluff, endow, etc. And, when your date shows up looking for Andy Garcia and turns to find Andy Rooney, let us know what you say to keep her in the room!

On the other hand, if your realistic goal is to actually hook up with someone in real life, do not lie here. After all, they're more than likely to notice when they meet you whether you smoke or have kids or what your height, weight, and age are.

In the long run, it's better to be up front than seem like a liar. Sure, it may not be "fun" to compose the following line, "I'm 5' 2" and weigh 300 pounds." But, perhaps you can try and be a little creative. For instance, technically, "Petite love muffin with a couple of extra blueberries" says basically the same thing, but in a little better package.

ACCURATE ADDRESSES

This is another sticky one. But you've already worked up a great title and learned how to put a positive spin on the fact that you're a two-headed swamp creature, so this should be no trouble at all. Naturally, another pertinent aspect to most personal ads is "location, location, location."

Of course, if you're taking an ad out in your local paper (did we mention trying the bar scene first?), this is a no-brainer. However, with the rise of the Internet and the thousands of personal ad sites out there clamoring for your business, the World Wide Web needs a few more specifics first.

But, again, not too many. For instance, if you live in Kalamazoo, Michigan, take a few extra minutes, haul out a map, and pen your location as "just outside of Detroit." That way, you won't have a hundred horny Hawaiians knocking down your door, but you won't put off a handful of hard-bodied Hoosiers who don't mind driving an extra couple of miles to meet you, either.

MIXED MESSAGES

All right. You've hooked them in, led them on, and told them (within a 1,000 mile radius, anyway) where you live. What's left? Only the most important part: the message of your personal ad. Just think of it as the plot of the novel of your life. But just exactly who are you? Jackie Collins? Stephen King? Danielle Steel? John Grisham? Dr. Seuss?

Naturally, when you're paying for ad space, you

don't want to write *War and Peace*. On the other hand, you want to come off as interesting as possible. Therefore, every word counts.

So take some time here and really focus. Be realistic. Who are you, anyway? Or who do you want to be? (Within reason.) More importantly, who do you want to meet? After all, if you concentrate on all those drama classes you took back in high school, as opposed to your current title as "Ms. Beer Guzzler '99," you're probably going to attract the wrong kind of guy. Okay, you'll actually be attracting the *right* kind of guy, just not the right kind for you.

A good rule of thumb is to keep things general. For instance, if you include the fact that you're a big fan of the Irish author of the month, you're giving out a lot of free information in the least amount of words. As in, you can read, have a sense of humor, pay attention to current trends, are a sucker for current trends, and don't really have a mind of your own. Okay, scratch that. Better say you're a big Stephen King fan. That should do it.

It's also a good idea to talk about what you want from this ad. To make friends? Get whipped and beaten while the soundtrack to *Evita* plays in the background? Fall in love? Meet someone to hang out with? Have sex with sheep while she watches?

Do you want something short term or long term? Do you just want to chit-chat? Or sit in painful silence while he tickles your toes with fresh beef jerky? Either way, no matter if it's true or not, don't, do not, write that you're desperate to get married and start a family right away.

Unless, that is, you don't *want* to get any responses back. On second thought, go ahead and include that part about marriage and kids. And, hey, don't forget the part about being desperate, clingy, and co-dependent. By all means, make sure that's in there. And, if it's at all possible, why not put it in your title. That way you'll have plenty of time to get back on the saddle and go check out the bar scene.

PERSONALS: REALITY BITES

It's Sunday morning and you've spent yet another weekend waiting by the phone, staring at the TV, and rearranging your sock drawer—again. Your sole contact with another human being was the delivery guy from Ping's take-out. The four pound Sunday paper lands with a thud on your doorstep and, spilling half of your first cup of coffee on the first twelve sections, the only readable print available to you are the last few pages of the Classifieds, otherwise known as the "personal ads."

"What the heck?" you think. You're alone. You're of legal age. And no one you care about will ever know that you spent a perfectly miserable Sunday morning and half a pot of coffee perusing through the personals. Not since you've closed all the blinds and lined the windows with Reynolds Wrap, anyway.

But now it's Sunday evening. The coffee's gone. You haven't eaten, bathed, or even napped.

TOP-5 REASONS TO WRITE A PERSONAL AD:

5.) The warden just approved your request for more free time.

4.) The nurses at the mental hospital are getting tired of playing "doctor."

3.) "Research" for next Sunday's sermon on cross dressing.

2.) The neighbor's dog told you to.

1.) You got tired of waiting for Jodie Foster to write back.

Yet your pulse is still pounding, your heart is racing, and your poor calves are sore from the incessant tapping of your over-excited feet.

You've found her. You just know it. The girl of your dreams, hidden right there for the whole world to see in Ad #312: *"SWF, 27, non-smoker, casual drinker, easy laugher. I'm a willowy blonde who's into reading, but not all the time. I like movies, but not foreign ones. I'm even into sports, indoor ones, that is. Only like-minded guys need apply. P. S. No freaks!"*

She's perfect. Just grand. What you've been waiting for all your life. Why, the only thing holding you back at all is the fact that she's placed a personal ad in the first place. But then, you were right there with her, reading each and every one of the 311 ads that preceded hers.

So who's the bigger freak? The willowy blonde who, probably on a dare from one of her similarly hot girlfriends, wrote *one* ad? Or you? The desperate guy who spent an entire unshaven, boxer short-clad Sunday morning, not to mention afternoon and evening, carefully combing six pages of fine newsprint for the love of your life?

After some cold lo mein and another cup of instant coffee, you count to ten, say a little prayer, write a similarly lighthearted and honest reply (*"Dear Ms. Willowy Blonde, you've found your part-time reading, foreign film hating, indoor sport loving non-freak here"*), find a stamp, and run out to the sidewalk to mail it to the newspaper's P. O. Box.

The next morning, however, an MSG and caffeine hangover is nothing compared with the regret you feel. Like Pee Wee Herman caught enjoying himself in the back row of a Florida movie theater, guilt racks your conventional brain and you're afraid that everyone at work, not to mention your mother, will know right away that you've done the unthinkable: answered a personal ad.

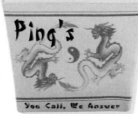

But your mother doesn't call and no one at work pays you any mind at all. And, when you finally race home after another mind-numbing day and see a big, fat zero on your answering

"Love is the answer, but while you're waiting for the answer, sex raises some pretty good questions."

– Woody Allen

machine, you're convinced that you have sunk lower than low. Not only have you answered a personal ad, but she's rejected you as well!

But then you remember the mail has to get to the paper, sit there for a while, and then get forwarded to your willowy blonde with the passion for paperbacks and domestic films. Breathing a sigh of relief, you spend the rest of the week alternately cursing the U. S. Postal Service and that willowy blonde from hell who won't even give your letter, or you for that matter, the time of day.

She calls the next Sunday, just as you've reached personal ad #385 in that week's paper—a SWF who loves archery, beat-up Fords, Cherry Garcia ice cream, and midget mud wrestling. Thank god, is all you can say, because by this time, of course, your willowy blonde has reached such an elevated status in your mind that it might as well be Princess Diana, or possibly Gwyneth Paltrow, on the other end of the line.

Between the sweat dripping from your forehead and her hoarse croak of a laugh that you somehow decipher as being sexy, you actually manage to make a date for later that evening at a bar equidistant between both of your places.

You change outfits seven times and brush your teeth five. You put on the Snoopy tie you told her you'd be wearing, not wanting to describe yourself and then have her find you wanting and not at all deserving of her willowy blondeness after all. Which, at this point, has now reached Uma Thurman proportions to you.

You get there early, not even scoping out an escape route because you know that this is it,

she's the one, she's chosen you and you are no doubt lucky with a capital "L."

She walks in forty minutes later smoking a cigarette (lie #1), at least six years older than thirty-seven, let alone twenty-seven (lie #2), and she's not so much willowy as she is winnow-y (as in horse, lie #3). And the only blonde on her head came out of a bottle, several months ago, judging from her black roots (lie #4).

Still, you've come this far and stand up, very gentlemanly, and hand her the pink carnation you bought from the flower girl half an hour earlier. She thanks you in a voice that would scare most professional wrestlers and instantly orders a scotch on the rocks, not exactly a "casual" drink, even for the cast of *Swingers* (lie #5).

Stunned into subdued silence, you let her fill most of the dead air between your barstools, which she does with tales of life in the trailer park and other hilarious stories of the redneck persuasion, half of which would embarrass Jeff Foxworthy.

When she runs out of whiskey-soaked ruminations on how many episodes of *Cops* she's personally been in, she entertains you with quickly crafted popcorn animals built from the bowl full of untouched kernels between you.

For glue she uses spit, her mortar is margarita salt, and by the time she has a zoo full of hot, buttered creature creations you realize why there are so many jokes, comics, funnies, and horror movies about personal ads: They're all true.

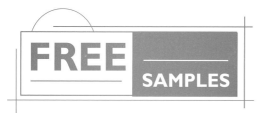

FREE SAMPLES

Wondering how your own personal ads stack up against the rest of the writing world? Here are a few samples culled from a variety of real personal ads posted in newspapers, newsletters, magazines, and the Internet. Although this section should not require a warning, here's one anyway: These ads are not supposed to get you excited or serve as templates for your own future personal ads. If they inspire either behavior, you might require something else that's also personal—therapy:

PICKY, PICKY!

"I like eating mayonnaise and peanut butter sandwiches in the rain, watching *Barney Miller* reruns, peeing on birds in the park, and licking strangers on the subway; you eat beets raw, have climbed Kilimanjaro, and sweat freely and often. Must wear size five shoes."

'NUFF SAID!

"Minimalist seeks woman."

SEXY SACRIFICE

"Patriarch of up-and-coming religion seeks altar girl with props."

SPICY SUDS

"Three-toed mango peeler searching for wicked lesbian infielder. Like screaming and marking territory with urine? Let's make banana enchiladas together in my bathtub. You bring the salsa."

AAA = Actual Ad Acronyms:

BBW = Big Beautiful Woman
BIF = Bisexual Female
CPL = Couple
Dom = Dominant
DBF = Divorced Black Female
DBM = Divorced Black Male
DDF = Drug and Disease Free
DWF = Divorced White Female
DWM = Divorced White Male
GBF = Gay Black Female
GBM = Gay Black Male
GWF = Gay White Female
GWM = Gay White Male
ISO = In Search Of
LTR = Long Term Relationship
MBF = Married Black Female
MBM = Married Black Male
MWF = Married White Female
MWM = Married White Male
Sub = Submissive
SBF = Single Black Female
SBM = Single Black Male
SWF = Single White Female
SWM = Single White Male
TS = Transsexual
TV = Transvestite

TURNING OVER A NEW LEAF

"Jane no good, Cheetah stinks. Tarzan seeks swinging GM to be the lord of his jungle."

GREAT SEXPECTATIONS

"SWM, old, fat, balding, many disgusting habits seeks SWF with money. Send pictures of your house, car, RV. This could be your lucky day."

OPPOSITES ATTRACT

"Hideous-looking, obese, smelly, ill-tempered, lazy, cowardly, chronic, and a complete liar seeks total opposite."

TRUE ROMANCE VS. TRUE CRIME

"Hello, I am Neil, 52-years old and single. I have a 12-year-old daughter that is my own, however, my former wife disappeared with her two years ago somewhere in the Philippines. I am an insurance agent and sold to myself large amounts of life insurance, which is very important, in that I now have a spreading prostate cancer that is expected to kill me within three years! #1715."

SOMEBODY GET BILL COSBY

"JELLO BOY—SWM who likes to slowly fold canned fruit into Jell-O, seeks female partner for distinctly American activities. Dirty pigeons need not respond. Teleclub Ext. 40485."

RACY RECIPE

"Mix on the Beach: Mix 1970 SWM, Vodka, Hazel melon, Pineapple Blonde Juice, Raspberry Liqueur, Cranberry Juice. Shake with 20-30 oz. SF in ice in a tall glass. Drink casually only."

KICK THE TIRES!

"1970 GMC w/Jet Skis. Low mileage, custom paint, long sandy blonde graphics. 6'2" Lift. Bright hazel headlights will take 20-30 SF anywhere. E-mail for free test drive/ride."

DARING DUO

"Superboy seeks Clark Kent. Come fly with me."

CHAINSAW MATCHMAKER

"SWM into chainsaws and hockey masks seeks like-minded SWF. No weirdoes, please."

DOUGHNUT DILEMMA

"SWM seeks 300lb+ woman to sit and squash doughnuts on me. Box 1234."

DO YOU BELIEVE IN MAGIC?

"WF, 37, misses Sabbath circles and talking to other Pagans. New to area and want to hook up with like-minded individuals. Interested in Tarot, herbal healing, acoustic music, art, and magic. No kooks!"

BEAK AND BLUE

"Fed up with watersports? Constrained by traditional dominant-submissive roles? Try a more nurturing role: feed me like a baby pelican! Both sexes welcome. I supply the raw herring, you bring the big strap-on beak. No weirdoes."

TIJUANA TWOSOME

"Bitter, unsuccessful, balding, middle aged loser wallowing in an unending sea of inert, drooping loneliness looking for 24-year-old needy leech-like hanger-on to abuse with dull stories, tired sex, and Herb Alpert albums. Baby, you are my Tijuana Taxi."

CARNEY BLARNEY

"Angry, simple-minded, balding, partially blind ex-circus flipper boy with a passion for covering lovers in sour cream and gravy seeks exotic, heavily tattooed piercing fanatic, preferably hairy and stinky, either sex, for whippings, bizarre sex, and fashion consulting. No freaks."

"If all these sweet young things were laid end to end, I wouldn't be the slightest bit surprised."
— Dorothy Parker

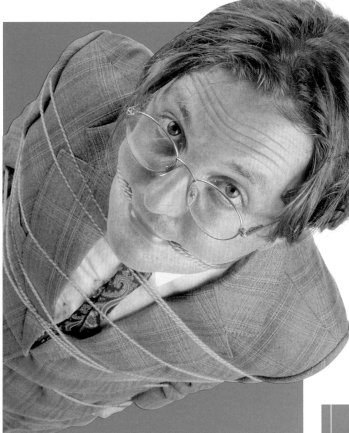

BOY TOY PLOY

"When I was thirty, my dates had to be young, slim, tall, handsome, rich, intelligent. Now I'm 64, they only have to know how to read and use the telephone!"

TYING THE KNOT?

"Submissive male seeks dominant female with extensive knowledge of knots."

COLD FEET

"There is a little place in the jumbled sock drawer of my heart where you match up all the pairs, throw out the ones with holes in them, and buy me some of those neat dressy ones with the weird black and red geometrical designs on them."

TOP-5 REASONS TO RESPOND TO A PERSONAL AD:

5.) Kills time while you're waiting in the unemployment line.

4.) You never realized you'd have so much free time on Death Row.

3.) Once the sermon for next Sunday is written, why not?

2.) Your other mail fraud schemes all fell through.

1.) Who needs a reason? You're a loser and you're lonely.

READING
BETWEEN
THE LOVE LINES

There is a line you cross. A mark in the sand. Your playful exploration of the local or even national personal ad sources becomes more grounded in reality. When, instead of being scattered across your kitchen table in a haphazard pile with last month's *Frederick's of Hollywood* catalog and the other junk mail you get every day, they actually get organized and thus take one step up the evolutionary ladder to your "home office." There, addresses are written down, stamps are purchased (in bulk), and sample ads are written and re-written on index cards with the help of handy dictionaries and thesauruses.

Of course, once you make the decision to delve into the murky world of personal ads, you are faced with a significant number of options as to where to find them. There is always the local paper, of course, which tends to weed out the more deranged ex-convicts or current prison and asylum escapees. In addition, there are the free trade papers offered in such fine establishments as, say, 7-11 and Circle K. There are also those pay services to consider, which take basic

personals one step further and throw in a video with the $99.99 "processing" fee. And, thanks to modern technology, there is now the Internet to help you find that kindred spirit even faster.

Despite the source you eventually choose, however, there are also the obvious code words of the personal ad vernacular, such as SWM, "single white male," or GM, which doesn't refer to a brand of American-made car, but instead a "gay male."

Obviously, these are the easy ones. Hidden deep inside the text of many a personal ad, however, are subtler, more "flexible" words that take a simple definition and tweak it to a very indefinable shape.

Take, for instance, the simple phrase, "Healthy, robust individual seeks same." Most of us see the word "healthy" and subconsciously picture the models on the covers of fitness magazines. Bikes slung over shoulders, thong bikinis, hiking boots, six-pack abs, etc. In the personal ad arena, however, "healthy" could mean anything from "barely breathing" to "actually able to get out of bed in the morning without the use of a crane."

Other adjectives become flexible in the personal ad arena as well. Perhaps you're a believer in that age-old motto, "opposites attract." Accordingly, you are seeking a powerful, strong, robust soulmate to round out your soft, sensitive, snoozy side. So you hunt through your chosen source of personal ads for vibrant descriptions. But which ones? Hmmm.

"blonde"

"healthy"

"robust"

"athletic"

"Adventurer." Ooh, that's a good one. How about "artistic?" That's nice, too. But before you get too excited, just remember where you're looking for these impressive individuals. For an "adventurer" in the peculiar world of personal ad lingo is simply someone who's had ten times the amount of sexual partners you have. While that "artistic" type you've been reading about is just putting a positive spin on the fact that he's unemployed and sells spray-painted hubcaps by the side of the road.

Get the picture?

It's not that the fractured folks who place personal ads are purposely trying to deceive you—okay, sure it is, but . . . it's sort of one of those "acceptable" deceptions that society may frown on but certainly doesn't condemn. Like "borrowing" extra packets of sugar with your small cup of convenience store coffee each morning so you never have to buy any for home. Or grabbing an extra newspaper for your boss when you buy one for yourself out of those vending machines.

In fact, most people who liberally sprinkle their personal ads with unrealistic traits and outright tall tales consider it just another form of "fluffing up" their reproductive resume.

Naturally, the personals are anything but immune to that ongoing battle of the sexes. Therefore, men and women tend to use quite a different set of adjectives to enhance their sparse strengths and hide their numerous weaknesses.

For instance, if a man includes his age in his ad, you can rest assured that, much like "dog years," this falsified figure is in some manner expressed in "personal ad years." Therefore, "40-ish" is simply a 52-year old man in search of a 25-year old woman. On the other hand, "twenty-something" usually means

162 IMA LOSER 26

x7

that some junior high school stud has a little too much time on his hands and can already turn a phrase.

Maybe your "dream man" has included the following impressive string of inflated "personal" traits in his audacious ad: "I consider myself athletic, reliable, and fun. I'm also honest, spiritual, and stable."

Translated into "reality speak," however, his crock of a curriculum vitae actually reads: "I regularly sit on the couch and watch ESPN, I'm punctual—give or take a few hours—and I'm always up for a little pizza and porn. I'm also a pathological liar who once went to church with his grandmother on Christmas Eve, as well as an occasional stalker, although I've never been convicted."

See how that works? And don't think it's just personality traits that get the pseudo-spin treatment. Personal ad writers are just as flexible with their physical traits as well. After all, any man who includes the "fact" that he is "good looking" is surely an arrogant, vain, narcissistic, mirror-worshipping jerk, while the semi-honest male who refers to himself as "distinguished looking" is most certainly fat, greasy, and balding.

Likewise, professions get just as malleable a personal ad treatment. Perhaps your dream man has written that he's a "professional." Technically, this could simply mean he owns a tie that his mom picked out before his 8th grade graduation ceremonies. Then again, maybe he's a "poet." Yeah, sure—whenever he remembers to bring a pen with him when visiting a public restroom stall!

Roses are red
Violets are blue
For a really good time
Call Sue – 555-1234

"But wait," you insist naively. "He also wrote that he was 'thoughtful,' 'virile,' and 'young at heart'! "

Human translation: a "thoughtful" personal ad patron will merely say "please" when demanding a beer. While "virile" simply means he can read three *Penthouse* Forums without passing out. And "young at heart?" Don't buy it. Everyone knows that this is the universal personal ad code for pedophile!

Conversely, if a female personal ad poet describes herself as "athletic," you can rest assured she's flat chested and has thighs the size of beer barrels. If she's "commitment-minded," be prepared to spend your first couple of dates at Home Depot picking out curtains for your long life together! If that womanly writer calls herself "romantic," she probably looks best by candlelight, preferably from across a ten-foot banquet table. And if she piques your interest with the declaration

that she's an "exotic beauty," you can guarantee her looks would scare even the Abominable Snowman!

Maybe her ad emphasizes the fact that she finds "communication important," (this means you'll be lucky getting a word in edgewise) and she stresses "friendship first," which can only mean that she's trying to live down her hard-earned reputation as a bonafide floozy. If she's "in transition," this simply means she needs a brand new sugar daddy to pay her bills. If she chooses to casually weave into her ad the fact that she's a "light drinker," rest assured she's bordering on becoming a full-time lush.

And be careful of that biggest of all personal punch lines, "young at heart." There's no doubt about this one fellas, she's a toothless crone.

So, now that you know the wacky world of personal ad poets isn't exactly full of Truthful Tommys or Literal Lucys, at least you'll be prepared when that "strapping, handsome hunk" you'd been planning on meeting turns out to be a chunky senior citizen the approximate shape and shade of a wedge of Swiss cheese whose claim of being "well-hung" is obviously referring to that 1957 clip-on necktie he's wearing.

Or is it?

TOP-5 EXCUSES TO GIVE YOUR BLIND DATE

5.) I have to pray to my fish.
4.) I need to spend more time with my toaster.
3.) I promised to help a friend lick stamps.
2.) I have some really hard words to look up.
1.) I have to check the freshness dates on my yogurt.

KEEPING AN EYE ON YOUR BLIND DATE

SUE'S STORY

He turned out, actually, to be a rather nice guy. You'd been worried about your first real blind date, but had been a little desperate after months of no dates at all, and had so done it anyway. Gulp!

Okay, so he's no Mel Gibson. But, like a swimmer who leapt off that dock called "25" a long time ago, you're halfway across the lake and well on your way to that distant dock on the other side, we'll call that one "35." So maybe your tastes have changed a little over the last few years.

You're quite a bit taller than he is, but looking up at all of those other guys you dated was getting a little tiresome. Flats are a lot more comfortable than heels anyway. You've got more hair than he does, but they're doing wonderful things with Extra-Strength Rogaine these days. Besides, when the two of you have been together long enough and feel a little more comfortable with each other, you're quite sure you'll be able to come up with a tactful way to broach the subject. His feet are smaller than yours, which is something a little new, but nothing major. Nothing huge.

The glass eye is a little bothersome, but who are you to judge other people's misfortunes? Still, it's hard to tell whether he's looking at you during dinner, or that little blonde at the next table. Oh well, just because his eye is artificial, doesn't mean it won't roam. He's a guy, after all.

After dinner, back at your place, the light jazz station is on, the candles are lit, and the box of wine he brought (okay, a little cheap, but a nice gesture, after all) is sweeter than soda but not quite as fattening. Either way, the evening is going well and you are finally thinking to yourself, "Wow. Could he be . . . okay? Could this . . . work out? Could he be it?"

"Look here," he says quietly, interrupting your blissful thoughts as you imagine the tiny feet of the plastic groom on your wedding cake stretching down an extra inch or two into that lattice-work frosting so that your proportions will be correct, "I've got something to show you."

Then, surprising you by not reaching for his zipper, he reaches instead for his jacket pocket and cups something small rather gingerly in his hand. "Close your eyes," he whispers, and you do. You feel his hand rest gently on your thigh for a minute before removing itself, rather gentlemanly, you decide.

"Now open them," he says with a smile. You do, and try not to wince when you see the extra glass eye he always keeps on him for emergencies resting on your thigh.

"See," he says playfully, "I've got my eye on you—literally."

Feigning laughter instead of shock, you realize suddenly that your dating days are finally drawing to a close.

Accordingly, you take another sip of your boxed wine and begin to seriously consider looking into becoming a mail-order bride.

> "I've had a perfectly wonderful evening. But this wasn't it."
> — Groucho Marx

Sound familiar? *Eerily* familiar? As in, "How did they get a hold of my personal diary?" familiar? Hmm, sounds like you've been on your share of blind dates lately. Well, at least you can take *some* comfort that you're not entirely alone. The fact is, we've all been on at least *one* blind date. Come on, fess up. You have too.

After all, the much bemoaned blind date is one of those relationship rites of passage we must all go through before earning our official "I'm a loser" badge in the Oh Boy (I'm Pathetic) Scouts. Like our mothers chaperoning us to the prom or forgetting our wallet at the snootiest restaurant in town, blind dates are just the really bad potholes along the superhighway of sex, dating, and relationships.

Fortunately, as an "almost" adult, you have the choice of whether or not to go on a blind date in the first place. After all, unless you have really forceful (as in, shotgun toting) friends, no one's actually forcing you to get dolled up and shave your legs on a Tuesday night just to go meet some prematurely balding car salesman at the local bowling alley for "two-for-one" drinks, a basket of cheese fries, and three glorious hours spent trying to desperately avoid his overzealous high-fives every time he knocks down more than two pins! But there does come a time in all our loveless lives when, out of sheer desperation, we are forced to undergo the inevitable blind date. And so, "in case of emergencies" only, here are a few tips that just might make the night at least slightly more pleasant (than getting a root canal, anyway).

The Shortest Blind Date in History

One boring weeknight there was a soft, feminine knock on my front door and I answered it to find my gorgeous babe of a centerfold neighbor standing there smiling at me in nothing but her bulging bathrobe and some fuzzy bunny slippers. Thinking that I was sleepwalking through my most decadent dream, the one where the two of us took a long, luxurious bubble bath together, I stood there dumbfounded, expecting to wake up at any minute.

"Would you like to go to a concert tonight?" she blurted, explaining that her boyfriend had stood her up at the very last minute, and that she now had two tickets, but no date. "They're awesome seats. Great band. It'll be one heck of a date, that's for sure!"

"I-I-I would I-I-love to go!" I stammered. Maybe it wasn't a dream after all, maybe I was merely sleepwalking.

"Super!" she replied. "Here you go. Enjoy the tickets and make sure you and your date have a blast!" She then handed over the tickets, waved good-bye, and padded off down the hall in those ridiculous slippers!

Talk about the shortest blind date in history.

Picky, Picky!

No matter what, make sure *you* pick the place. After all, the first tenet of any dating philosophy worth its salt is that you are the "catch" and that your fortunate date for the evening is the "lucky one." Now, with that in mind, try picking someplace you've always wanted to go but never have before.

Make it convenient for you. Who knows, maybe

there's a quaint little coffee shop right around the corner you've just quite never managed to venture into yet. Or a biker bar down the street that has free pool and great drink specials. How about the funky vegetarian restaurant that always smells tempting as you drive by after work?

This ploy is two pronged. Number one, by being stubborn and forcing your blind date's hand, you can often avoid the evening altogether. "Forget that," your insolent intended might scoff. "If she's already being this bull-headed, imagine what she'd be like if we started dating!"

On the other hand, if your date agrees willingly, he or she might not be as bad as you thought. Perhaps they're even interested in you for real! After all, you've made a pretty "picky" demand and they've acquiesced. Score one for you!

Win, Win!

Now that you've chosen the meeting place, it's time for the second part of the date. Okay, you've had the cinnamon cappuccino at the cozy coffee shop and haven't managed to lunge at each other. Or perhaps you've shared one of those drink specials (or two, or three) at the biker dive without getting inducted into the local chapter of the Hells Angels. Great. Super. On to the fun.

And that's the key: fun. Many blind dates start off on the wrong foot before either of you even get past, "Hello." Instead of planning on a regular, old, boring night of "dinner and a movie," why not have a little fun! Do something you'll be able to enjoy even if she's a complete and utter bore or he grinds his teeth whenever he's not speaking (which isn't often!).

An experimental play at the local college you've been meaning to attend but never quite found the courage to go to is a great idea. Or how about a concert at the local high school featuring scattershot, drum-heavy renditions of the century's greatest Broadway plays? Those pottery-painting places are great, and, even if the

date sucks, at least you'll have an oversize coffee mug or ceramic birdhouse as a souvenir.

As you can see, the goal here is to make your blind date a "win/win" situation. If the date completely sucks and the two of you have absolutely nothing in common (except perhaps your mutual loathing of each other), then at least you've taken in a great night of theater or basket weaving. Which is still a win. On the other hand, if you hit it off and end up igniting that oft heard of, rarely witnessed "spark," then great. You win *both* ways!

Excuses, Excuses!

Regardless of the place you've picked out or the winning strategy you've devised, always have a good excuse ready. Just in case. After all, that friendly biker bar could have gotten raided over the weekend or the high school band could have suddenly come down with a bad case of crabs. (You just never know about kids these days. Even band kids!)

So a good excuse is as integral a part of the blind date as is lipstick or Old Spice. This is where cell phones come in handy. Even if you don't own one, borrow one! Then arrange for someone to call you about thirty minutes after the date starts. Come on, you can make it that long, can't you? Okay, make it fifteen minutes.

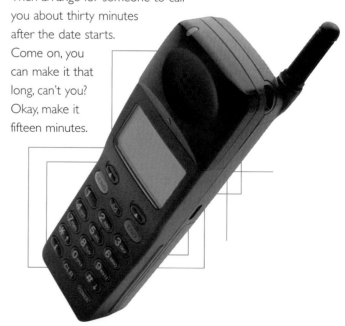

Either way, the person on the other end can be speaking pig Latin for all you care, just so long as a phone rings and offers you up the opportunity to say something sly and sinister, such as, "What? What? Grandma Madrigal passed away? Again?"

Hey, what Granny doesn't know won't hurt her, right? After all, she's probably been on her share of blind dates too.

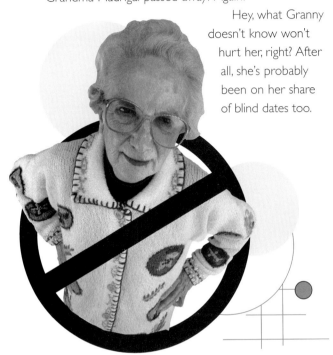

Precautions, Precautions!

Okay, okay, enough cynicism for one evening. Let's think positive for a change. (Jeez, all the good ones can't be taken, right? Right?) Now, considering the place you picked was cozy, the entertainment for the evening enjoyable, and the cell phone strategy wasn't necessary, chances are you're having a good blind date!

So what now? Well, this is where shaving your legs on a boring, old Tuesday night comes in handy. Only, don't stop there. Are your sheets a little dirty? Wash them. Not enough clean wine glasses in case you need a little "nightcap" so you can both get your second wind? Wash those too.

Have a bestseller or two on your coffee table. Cue up a few romantic CDs just in case. New candles are a nice touch. (So are new underwear. Wink, wink, nudge, nudge.) Hey, no one's suggesting you go all the way on your first date. Your first "blind date" no less.

But, after all, it was your choice to go on this blind date. What did you think would happen?

Disastrous Drive-in Dating Diet

It was my first blind date and I was really nervous. A mutual friend had set us up, and, just to avoid any huge surprises when we met, we'd exchanged "recent" pictures through our matchmaker. He was a total hunk and, I admit, I've been known to have my "naughty" side. Luckily, the latest retro rage in our town had resulted in a new drive-in theater downtown. I thought it would be a great place for our blind date. That way, if he was just a pretty face with no brain, we could enjoy the movie and not waste the whole night. But, if his brain matched his body and we hit it off, we could spend the evening…necking. Either way, I win.

He thought it was a great idea too and when he picked me up I got nothing but good vibes off of him. We had comfortable small talk on the way there, he paid for the movie and the snacks, and we both settled in for a few minutes of the movie before I made my first move. When I did, he reciprocated by caressing my thirty-year old stomach. In the sexiest voice I'd ever heard, he said, "Oh, how sweet. You brought along a spare tire in case I get a flat…"

I'd never been more embarrassed, and our blind date ended right there. I threw a total hissy fit and ate the whole tub of popcorn on the way home. I'm no Ally McBeal, but I'm no Dom DeLuise either. What do guys expect these days? Isn't there anyone out there who likes a girl with a little meat on her bones?

3
LOVE AT FIRST (WEB) SITE

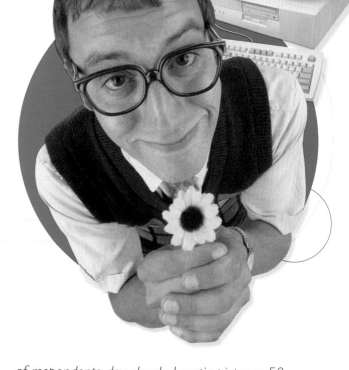

Could it be "love at first byte?" The rapidly expanding, ever-sophisticated Internet market presents a new use for clicking keyboards and well-worn mousepads: real-time romance. Think about it. Nothing happens. Everything happens. Cybertalk and Cyberwalk, Cyberguys and Cyberchicks, Cybergay and Cyberstraight, Cyberlove and Cybersplit. Cyberhope and Cybergloom—and you never have to leave your room.

Cyberspace: that tricky, sticky virtual world where everything from pickled herring to porn is only a double-click away. No one owns it, no one controls it, but we all use it. And, for some of us, we're using it to find a mate. Or, at least, someone to mate with.

While the perception may be that every single one of your hipper, cooler, more with-it friends is currently engaged in some tawdry form of online dating, erotic e-mail exchange, or cybersex, the fact is that such hearty souls are still in the matrix minority. According to Survey.Net, an Internet polling company, only ten percent of respondents actually placed an online personal ad, yet eleven percent admit to replying to a personal ad. But twelve percent of people surveyed actually had sex with someone they met online.

The majority of recorded online sexual behavior is decidedly "one-handed": 56 percent

of respondents downloaded erotic pictures, 50 percent read online sex stories, and 33 percent of respondents masturbated while online!

What happens when one lonely guy finds the chat-room cutie of his dreams, only to find that his hottie is actually a hunk? Or how about the hot-wired hottie whose hard-drive hunk turns out to be a cyberstalker in disguise? Click forward.

AMOROUS ADVENTURES IN CYBER DATING

Oh, the cyber chat room, that warm, fuzzy glow on your computer screen full of funky names like "Dial-Up Diva" and "Roger-Rabbit-69," where you can say anything and, more important, be anything you want, hope, or dream of being. Whether it be a CEO of your own dot.com, an entrepreneur with eighty-five inventions under your belt, or a buff beach bunny with perfect skin and measurements to induce metabolic meltdown, the Internet now affords any and all the ability to assume a whole other identity.

For who's to know if you're actually a pizza delivery boy driving your parents' car while sitting on a phone book or a salesgirl down at Spencer's who needs a foot stool to reach the cash register? And, after all, who cares?

If chat rooms are the Internet's answer to tall tales and fish stories told by the virtual campfire, then screen names must be the cyber-equivalent of cucumber-lined Levi's and tissue-stuffed wonderbras. What else can you assume? After all, every single name crowded into that steamy, sweaty chat room alludes to supremely masculine members (Power Tool) or well-endowed measurements (Truck Flap Model), usually accompanied by so-called "actual" measurements, which, if they were all to be believed, would make America the undisputed home to every well-hung, pinup-worthy hard-body on the entire planet.

Of course, there is no moment of truth more skin-crawlingly creepy or filled with hopeful (some cynics would say naïve) anticipation than meeting a chat room romance live and in person for the very first time—outside of cyberspace, that is. What do you wear to meet a self-proclaimed "perfect 10" when you are a simple single digit on the low end of the scale? Will you be able to be as pithy, sexy, or romantic (depending on the situation) as you were back in the chat room, where coy, witty, or ribald statements were scribbled out on scrap paper before being typed in on the keyboard? And what if those imported French lifts you'll need to place in your shoes so that you can live up to your statuesque proportions don't arrive in time?

To avoid such hard-drive hi-jinx, you must take a few simple precautions when combing today's cornucopia of chat-rooms.

poems and then reading them to appreciative women. Hmm, sounds good. But if this grammar guru actually said, "I luvs to red, writ, and relly, relly luvs to writ down them durty songets and then reds them in the crapper to ya" chances are he might not be the next author on *The New York Times* best-seller list.

Sure, a few typos are okay, but come on!

SLOW AND STEADY WINS THE RACE

Certainly, chat rooms can be a completely innocent place to flirt, wink, and nudge your way through an otherwise boring weeknight. And that's fine. But if you want to extend your chat room conversation into a weekend activity that actually takes place live and in person, why rush it? Does it just absolutely, positively *have* to be this coming weekend?

After all, for most Net heads, finding the right chat room takes nights and nights, if not weeks and weeks, of dedicated surfing. So if it's taken you this long to find the right chat room, let alone the right chat cat, surely you can wait until next weekend to meet. This is a good way to test a newcomer's intentions, as well. If your new friend, ScarlettIDareYa, insists that it's either "this weekend or nothing," then chances are he's just another shady businessman looking for a quick romp while using the handy dataport down at the local motel. (Either that, or a crafty con on an extremely liberal work release program.)

So there's no harm, no foul in missing out on that "golden opportunity" anyway. If, on the other hand, your digital date agrees with you, maybe he is on the up and up after all. And if he isn't, you've just earned yourself an extra week to find out!

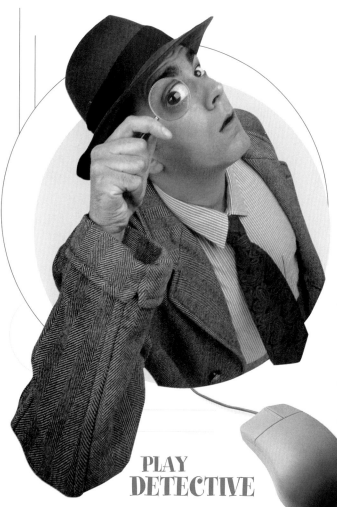

PLAY DETECTIVE

Just because you're sitting down, wearing baggy pajamas, and munching contentedly on stale Pringles doesn't mean you should let your guard down when cruising a chat room. Okay, sure, it's easier to believe everything you read on that glowing computer screen. And, if you're going there just to "screen name" watch, fine. Watch away.

But if you're looking for love, or at the very least, a little lust, then try and read between the lines a little. Say you've started conversing with a particularly friendly fellow, who goes by the screen name BookWorm, and he's just invited you to "join him" in a quieter chat room without the "meat market" overtones of the one you just met each other in. Okay. Fine. So far, so good.

But as you begin sharing information about each other, pay attention. BookWorm says he's an avid reader, loves to write, and especially enjoys writing love

"The perfect love affair is one which is conducted entirely by post."

—George Bernard Shaw

BE an ENIGMA UNTO YOURSELF

As you're chatting, try to be a little mysterious. After all, why buy the cow when you can get the milk for free? (Whoops, wrong kind of chatting.) Anyway, reality is a tenuous balloon in any chat room, so why wade in right away with the fact that your last three boyfriends died tragic deaths right after breaking up with you? (Unless you're trying to get rid of your new cyberpal, that is.)

Let him ask you questions and, when he does, give him cryptic answers. Don't be obtuse, but try not to be so forthcoming. After all, everyone "expects" to hear a little positive spin when they're in a chat room. That's what they're for.

So go ahead, spice things up a little. The great thing about chat rooms is their anonymity. Your new friend doesn't know you're the shyest thing since carved stone. Be free! Let your inner you come out, just not all at once.

JUST the FACTS, SIR!

To keep your feet on the ground in any chat room romance, keep a notepad handy by your keyboard. Jot down specifics you think might be "iffy." His 1,000-foot yacht, for instance. If it keeps getting smaller, this might be an eventual red flag that what he really owns is a rusted out shrimp skiff. Remember that it's all in the details.

If he says he's a world class sommelier but can't even suggest what type of wine you might enjoy with a nice Porterhouse, chances are he's not being entirely truthful. On the other hand, even if he does suggest the appropriate wine with the appropriate meal, that could just mean he's got *The Buzz On Wine* open in front of him.

So how does one win in this chat room of love? Simple: don't fall for the hype! The Internet is great. The World Wide Web is wondrous. But it's not an instant

answer to your soul-searching questions of the heart. Treat it like you would a blind date (a *really* blind date) or a guy you've heard about from a friend of a friend. Take it slow, nice and easy, pay attention, stay focused and, just like anything else, don't rush into anything.

Words are just that, words. And they can only say so much. It may sound corny, but listen to your heart. If that pounding muscle is screaming out questions like, "If this guy's so rich, gorgeous, intelligent, and sought-after, what's he doing in this lousy chat room?" Chances are your brain will catch up sooner or later. Just try and wait until then to make any important decisions!

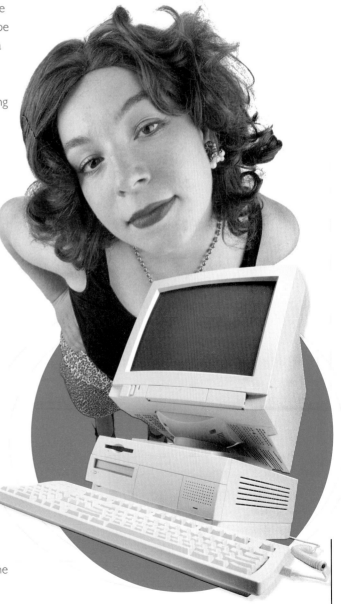

CYBER CONFESSION:
"COOPED" UP IN CYBERSPACE

I should have known better than to go into one of those "adult-themed" chat rooms. But it had been so long in between dates, I guess I'd gotten a little desperate. Amazingly, I found a kindred soul who said she "hated" having to resort to meeting people this way. We sort of paired off and she invited me to a less crowded "room," where we "talked" for hours. Still, I wasn't surprised when she didn't want to exchange phone numbers with me and actually talk for real. It's a cruel world out there, and I assumed she'd been burned once too often.

However, because of our intense "bond," she agreed to meet me that weekend at a bar of her choosing. Naturally, this gave me a couple of days to mull over my decision to actually meet this enchanting stranger. After all, the bar was foreign to me and I wasn't too sure about the neighborhood it was located in, either. But the more I thought of reasons why not to go, the more my heart, and loins, insisted I try something new and unique. After all, whatever I'd been doing for the past year and a half sure hadn't been working.

Naturally, I got "duded up" and went, despite my inner fears. I had a hard time finding the place and, naively, assumed that The Chicken Coop was just another western-themed bar. After all, there sure were a lot of guys in cowboy hats inside. Of course, there were all kinds of guys inside wearing all kinds of other hats too: biker helmets, baseball caps, and berets. There were even one or two guys wearing hats Princess Diana would have been proud of.

Sure enough, the only thing western about The Chicken Coop was its patrons undying love of leather chaps. My "date" scooped me up in a bear hug and ordered me a beer before I could retreat from *his* viselike grip. Somehow, I managed to escape his tentacles and land safely on a barstool next to him.

"You're not serious," I said, too shocked to form more words than the bare minimum. "You told me you were blonde, stacked, and built like a brick house."

"Dude," said the fifty-year old businessman who obviously "fancied" himself the hottest boy-toy in town. "I am blond, stacked, and built like a brick house —where it counts."

I looked at the gray-haired, pasty-faced imposter across from me and sipped my imported beer. Not only had he duped me into thinking he was the "girl" of my dreams, but he didn't even make such a great argument for luring me over to his "side." I mean, even if I was bi-curious, was a guy who reminded me more of my dad than my sugar-daddy supposed to turn me into a switch-hitter?

Needless to say, the next time I risk meeting someone from a chat room face to face, I'm getting a picture first. At least that way, I can make sure it's worth my while to head down to The Chicken Coop first.

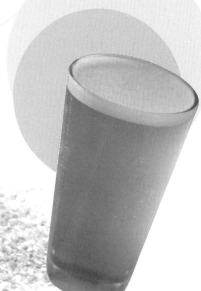

CYBER CONFESSION: AWOL ON AOL

I met a girl on one of the Internet dating sites on AOL. We e-mailed for a while and finally decided to meet. Since neither of us wanted to end up in a true-crime book, we followed all of the cyber-dating advice and met at a public place. As a true cyber-geek, I showed up forty minutes early just to scope the place out and make sure it wasn't some secret meeting point for the Ku Klux Klan.

Actually, it turned out to be one of those little neighborhood coffee bars with funky armchairs and cozy couches. I felt just like I was on the set of *Friends*.

Okay, so I'm no Joey. I'm not even Chandler. Hey, even Ross is a stud compared to me. But I'm no Quasimodo, either.

TOP-5 INTERNET SITES TO AVOID WHEN WEB SURFING ALONE AT NIGHT

5 icanseeyou.com

4 stalker.org

3 recentparolee.com

2 theguyunderyourbed.net

1 alreadyinsideyourhouse.org

And it's not exactly like I'd described myself as a cross between Brad Pitt and Tom Cruise. I think, in one of our mutual e-mails, I'd told my cyber-blind date that I was "distinctive looking."

Anyway, I sat there like an idiot for the next three hours with a yellow carnation in my pocket waiting for her to show up. She never did. I spent $15 on yuppie coffee and couldn't sleep for the rest of the night. Naturally, surfing the Internet at 4 a.m., still wired, I checked my e-mail to find a terse message from my would-be Wonder Woman: "Dear Mr. Distinctive Looking, nice try. I sat in the Laundromat across the street from our bar to get a better look at you before we met. At first, I was hoping the geek in the glasses and stripes and plaids wearing a yellow carnation in his pocket protector was a coincidence. No such luck. Next time save us both the hassle and tell the truth. You're not distinctive looking…you're disgusting!"

It really hurt my feelings, but it taught me a great lesson: cyber-blind-dating may be convenient, but it can also be pretty cruel.

CYBER CONFESSION:
BLIND DATE'S
XENA SHRINE?

I met this girl online, and she seemed like a total sweetheart. We moved to a more "private" chat-room, if there is such a thing, and exchanged phone numbers. When she called, I was totally blown away. She had the sexiest voice I'd ever heard. I know you hear horror stories about chat room hook-ups turning out to be total trolls and hags, but I didn't even care. With a voice as sexy as hers, I could just close my eyes and imagine a body to match.

Eagerly, I set up a date and was surprised when she invited me to her apartment. Most of the time people agree to meet somewhere. Still, when she was talking, I could hardly say, "no." I drove to her place that Friday and picked up Chinese food and beer on the way over. When she answered the door, I was stunned to see a total hottie staring back!

Everything was going great. Then I had to ruin everything by asking to use the bathroom, which just happened to be located in her bedroom. On the way, I noticed an actual shrine to *Xena: Warrior Princess*. I mean, this thing had it all: posters, 8 x 10 glossies, candles, bows and arrows, plastic swords, and even toy horses!

After that, it was all downhill. She got a headache from the MSG in the Chinese food and I drank too much beer. She kept dropping tiny hints about her sexuality, and I got the distinct feeling that I was a first-time experiment of the male persuasion that had gone very, very wrong. Her cold feet were obvious and I left before she made a big mistake. The funny thing is, she called me the next day and we went out and had a great time. Both of us were relaxed, now that we both knew where she stood. We've been friends ever since.

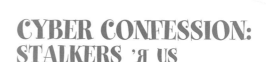

CYBER CONFESSION:
STALKERS 'R US

You might think that, as a freelance photographer, my dating dance card is pretty much always full. After all, my job is to run around all day taking snapshots of hunky, half-naked male models who hand me their phone numbers at the end of each shoot. Right? More like "yeah, right!" In reality, I take more pictures of flooded basements (for insurance reasons) and pet dogs (for God knows what reasons) than I do actual human beings, let alone macho male models.

So, like everyone else in this modern age, I spend my fair share of time cruising the singles' chat rooms late at night after the film's developed and my own dogs are asleep. And even though such actions might sound drastically desperate, I'm actually quite careful.

Which is why I was so surprised when what happened actually happened.

I'd "met" this guy in one of my favorite, cleanest, safest (or so I thought) dating chat rooms. For starters, he had one of the more "normal" screen names (as opposed to, say, "Edsmalldick" or "MaleGod#1"): JustJoe. JustJoe said he was a carpenter and loved working with his hands. (Never a bad thing, from my point of view. After all, Harrison Ford started out as a carpenter too!) He liked going to movies and eating at hot dog stands. Both of which appealed to me after dating my share of snooty snobs who look down on you if you don't know what kind of imported wine to drink with your escargot.

Eventually, after several long nights spent baring our souls all over our monitors, we took that all important first step and exchanged phone numbers. And so began the nightmare! From that evening on, almost as soon as I got offline, my phone started ringing and never stopped. And not with whispered sweet nothings, requests for dates, or even heavy breathing! It would ring, I'd pick it up and hear that spooky silence that we single girls living alone just *love* to hear. For the rest of that week, the phone rang non-stop, morning, noon, and night.

I know what you're thinking, "so just change your number!" Yeah, really? As a freelancer, all of my work comes over the phone lines. New work, old acquaintances, people who have seen my number on business cards at the back of their wallets or in that "cheap" classified ad in the paper I spend $15 a week on! Changing my number was a big, big step.

Eventually, however, it was a step I had to take. After all, I could hardly take professional photos without a decent night's sleep! I estimate my one (and only) chat room "rendezvous" cost me hundreds of dollars in lost business. And I never even met the guy. Naturally, when I called "his" number, all I got was the local Pizza Hut!

And don't think I didn't take advantage of that. I may have lost money, but I sure gained weight.

GOT MALE! (OR FEMALE!)

Although an e-mail address still doesn't have the same private overtones as an actual phone number or "snail mail" address, it nonetheless signifies a semi-significant relationship of some sort.

"I can't believe you stood me up for the Lilith Fair concert," a girlfriend might say, obviously hurt. "Didn't you get my e-mail?"

"Nooooo," the boyfriend may reply, feigning shock before adding quickly (not to mention cleverly), "but then, you know those damn e-mail servers."

In many ways, e-mail has given modern singles a brand new, not to mention convenient, buffer zone, affording them ample time to decide whether to pass on a real, non-pizza parlor phone number or start up an entirely new e-mail account with another Internet provider instead.

Besides, everyone knows that writing a note is the cheap way out of, or into, any relationship. The hit film *Shakespeare in Love* notwithstanding, does anyone actually believe the bard really spoke like that? Out loud? All the time? Even when hungover after a heavy night of too much mead or all of those feather and ink fumes?

Certainly notteth.

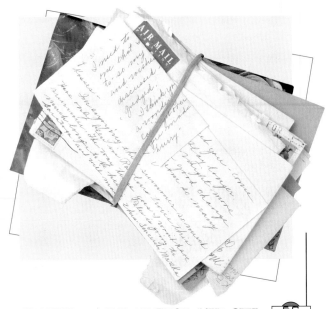

TOP-5 E-MAIL SUBJECT HEADINGS YOU NEVER WANT TO READ

5 RE: your upcoming audit

4 Greetings from Sing Sing!

3 RE: your daughter's recent herpes test

2 From the laptop of Theodore Kaczynski

1 Congratulations! Your naked pictures are now posted on bigass.com

with his 'software' and knows how to do more than just tinker around with my hard drive. :(Jane."

Hitting "send" isn't even as hard as licking that old-fashioned stamp and walking down to the corner mailbox, which always provided ample time for second thoughts anyway. If we can now buy books, CDs, and even stocks with the click of a button, why not end a messy relationship, too?

Naturally, this emotionless e-mail solution can just as easily backfire if you're not careful. Especially when drinking is involved. After all, computers and solitary confinement often go hand in hand. Maybe it's Wednesday evening (*late* Wednesday evening). It's been a hard week. Okay, half a week. You've been listening to the Indigo Girls and sipping a heady '98 Shiraz all night while searching dirty keywords on Yahoo! when, suddenly, you run across that studly new guy in Accounting's

The fact is, it's simply easier to "write" a "so-long sonnet" or, in modern language, a "Dear John" letter than to go through an actual, "Hey, uhm, John, listen. Why don't you sit down," confrontation in person at the local tavern, where dirty martinis (not to mention dirty punches) could easily be thrown.

"Dear John," one might click away instead, a company laptop perched on one's soon-to-be single-again lap as the subway lurches forward toward an inevitably funky bachelorette loft. "By the time you get this, we will be over, through, kaput. Thanks for the good times, but I've given my e-mail address to a real man—one who doesn't have quite so many problems (can you say, oxymoron?) e-mail address in the company newsletter.

Whoa, Nellie! A few more sips of wine, a couple of passionate, longing, soulful sentences and you've got yourself quite a tempting message on your glowing computer monitor. It's simply scandalous, really, the way you can rhyme so many words with "horny" and not even crack a thesaurus!

Well, fortunately, you'd never actually "send" such a torrid tome. And, since you're not, why not add a few more lascivious limericks and, what the heck, go ahead and sign it, too. It's all just fun and games anyway and, whoops, look out for that wine bottle as you go to fan your sensual self. Wouldn't want it to tip over just so and fall onto your laptop, and, holy smokes, what are the odds the lip of the bottle would double-click the mouse that way?

Hey. Whoa. What the—why is there a tiny little window in the middle of your screen flashing those five little words that will make it impossible for you to go to work for the rest of the week (if ever again): Your mail has been sent!

Hmm, on second thought, maybe "snail mail" isn't so bad after all.

BUDDY LIST BLUES

Say what you want about AOL, but the McDonald's of Internet providers was smart enough to call its list of friends who might be online at the same time as you a "buddy list," and not a "one-night stand bordering on a real relationship sometime in the near future" list. Such a decision, one assumes, was not arrived at solely as a "space conservation" issue, either.

You know what a "buddy list" is, right? (If you don't, consider yourself one of the lucky ones!) A "buddy list" is a feature offered by AOL that allows you to type in a list of your best friend's screen names: SpaceBoy3, PrincessPam, DirtyDogDan, PartyGirl911, etc. This way, when you're online checking your e-mail, running a search engine, or just surfing for single male underwear models, you can see if your friends are online at the same time.

For instance, say it's late Thursday night, you're busy e-mailing yourself at work a couple of files from your day spent "telecommuting" from home. You've been slogging through tiresome forecast charts, pie graphs, market projections, etc. when, suddenly, out of nowhere, a cute little "ding" announces that your favorite buddy of all, MrMojo, has just logged on to his AOL account three miles away in his very own sweat sock smelly den.

And, if you have been kind enough to supply MrMojo with your screen name, HunkAlert, and he has been focused enough to add you to *his* buddy list, the two of you are in business.

"What's happening?" you can type into the handy little "buddy box" in the left corner of your screen. Hit "enter" and your message is instantly transported to his buddy box across town.

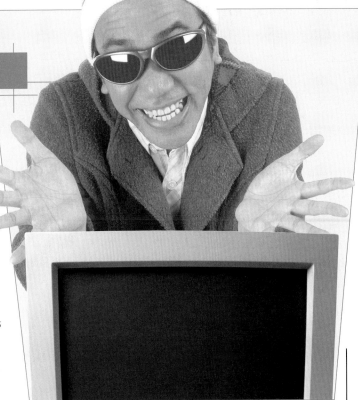

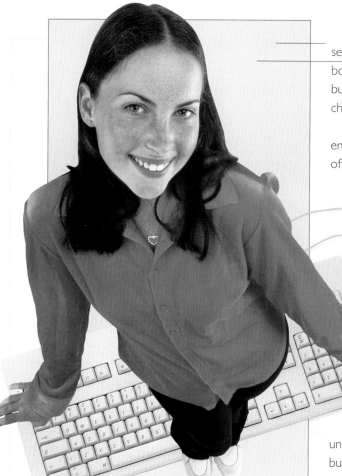

Of course, when the buddies are of the opposite sex, things tend to heat up a bit. Say it's the same boring weeknight and, miracle of miracles, your new buddy from work, SusieStockbroker, chimes in with her charming "ding."

"What's cooking, doll?" she might type into her empty buddy box. "Can't believe you weren't in the office today. I've got so much dirt to dish, you won't believe it. Now, where to begin."

And, as your own buddy box fills with bold tales of office romance and secretary shenanigans, you could spend all night just staring at her clever turn of phrase and choice of work-related words.

Naturally, it helps to picture her gorgeous, long gams and flowing auburn hair while you're at it.

Somehow AOL must have known that getting your name added to one of these ever-elusive lists was the cyber-equivalent of "forgetting" your toothbrush, lucky thong underwear, or left earring at your "friend who's a boy, but not quite a boyfriend's" house.

In many ways, considering the information highway we're all currently hitchhiking on, the "buddy list" may well be one of the last remaining bastions of cyber-privacy.

For while e-mail addresses can be bought or sold, deleted or spammed, zapped with a virus or "top-ten" listed to death, creating a buddy list takes an actual extra, physical step that many cyber-singles today aren't quite willing to take just yet.

Perhaps it's simply that they've been "buddy burned" once or twice. For, in the rush and gush of a fledgling romance, it's so easy to type in a simple, clever screen name and be done with it.

It's even a fun, pleasant surprise to hear that little "ding" and then see your new buddy's address pop up in a convenient little screen with a jaunty message like "what's up, little lady?" or "how they hangin'?"

Of course, don't be fooled by the lighthearted little moniker. For while "buddy" may sound simply chummy, in cyber reality, it can be as serious as a one-

Just like that! No messy looking up his screen name in your cyber address book. No writing an e-mail and having to hit send while you wait for the spell-check program to run because you forgot how to turn it off months ago. No waiting several minutes for him to get your e-mail, read it, and then reply with one of his own.

It's instant, it's fast, and—look, he's already written you back!

MrMojo: "Not much, just surfing the Web, trying to find the cheapest airfare on a couple of tickets to San Francisco."

Of course, when it's approaching midnight and MrMojo is still explaining, in minute detail, every last second of his planned California itinerary, you might regret adding him to your buddy list in the first place. Still, buddies are buddies.

night stand or even a three-month fling. To avoid being "buddy burned," here are a few general rules to follow when adding, or deleting, a new buddy name.

Don't be a Buddy Slut

Just because it's a simple little screen name or two, don't be slutty with your buddy. Exchanging e-mail addresses with a guy you've just met in a lovely little coffee shop downtown is one thing. If you're doing it to be polite and get rid of the guy, you can always claim you spilled coffee all over it after he left. Or, if that fails and he actually e-mails you, you can always claim you hit "delete" instead of "send" if you ever see him again, and he asks why you never e-mailed him back. (See how easy it is to be a cyber liar?)

But buddy lists are another matter altogether. For one thing, if he adds your screen name to his buddy list, he can actually see when you're online. No, really.

TOP-5 SIGNS YOU'RE ADDICTED TO THE INTERNET

5 You actually know what URL stands for.

4 If it weren't for Pop-Tarts, you'd starve to death.

3 Your den smells worse than your college dorm did.

2 You've named your mouse.

1 You learned of your impending divorce from your spouse's Web page.

Another little box, on the other side of your screen, reveals a list of "Buddies online." And you'll be in it!

Not that we're saying he'll be lurking online at all hours of the day and night, grinning eerily in the blue monitor light over a fresh pot of coffee while drool forms in the corner of his mouth and his hands shake, but if he is, you're going to get caught logging on sooner or later. Trust us.

He'll hear that little "ding," see your cleverly perky screen name, and boom. Before you know it, your buddy box is full of clever, frisky, instant messages:

Cyberstalker: "Feeling lucky?"

Cyberstalker: "How fast can you type? I'd love to be your keyboard right now—"

Cyberstalker: "Care to use my face as a mousepad?"

Cyberstalker: "Ever tried cybersex before?"

And, try as you might to ignore it, the way those instant messages keep adding up, along with their accompanying, now annoying, "dings," you might as well have invited a high school band into your home office. And that's just with one "buddy!" Imagine what could conceivably happen if you've been particularly "easy" with your screen name, handing it out to every Tom, Dick, and Scary in the office.

Now, how fast did you say you could type?

Be a Multiple

Of course, if you just can't say "no" to all those potential buddies out there, investigate your Internet provider's policy on screen names. Many allow you to have several e-mail accounts and even more screen names. Take advantage of these liberal policies and start signing on with a different screen name. Sure, it's a pain in the butt, but it's better than wearing earplugs every time you sign on and taping an index card over your buddy box! Besides, once you get used to it, you'll forget all about your "former cyber self" and embrace the new one.

And, if you don't, wait a while. The nice thing about the Internet is its speed. No, we're not talking about how quickly those "naked" pictures of "Brad Pitt" download. But your former buddy, having spent

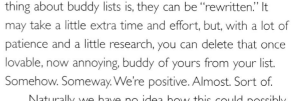

thing about buddy lists is, they can be "rewritten." It may take a little extra time and effort, but, with a lot of patience and a little research, you can delete that once lovable, now annoying, buddy of yours from your list. Somehow. Someway. We're positive. Almost. Sort of.

Naturally, we have no idea how this could possibly be done. (This is a book on Sex, Dating, & Relationships, after all. Not Cobol, Unix, & Hypertext!) But, rest assured, it can be done. And, if not just now, it certainly will be able to be done in the near future. Of that we're quite sure. Until then, of course, you're stuck with your buddy for the time being. (Hey, don't blame us. We told you not to be a buddy slut!)

Excuses, Excuses!

Of course, if you don't own a set of earplugs, have to use the Internet for a total of six hours each and every evening, and still can't figure out how to add or delete bothersome buddies from your list, you can always fall back on that bastion of all things dating: excuses.

"How come you never wrote me back last night?" your burned buddy might ask the next morning from three cubicles over. "And don't lie, my buddy box told me you were online!"

"Actually," you might reply, "I did log on, but then, see, I had some soup on the burner, and it overflowed and started a small blaze and the fire department got involved and, it was just a mess. I guess I forgot to log off."

Naturally, you can probably come up with something a little better than that. Just as long as you come up with something. Of course, if all else fails, you can always buy a new computer.

Hey, it's better than moving. Right?

numerous sleepless nights just waiting for the chance to inundate your buddy box with a fresh batch of pseudo-sexy instant messages, will probably tire of the game before too long.

Yes, though it's hard to admit, your former buddy will most likely move on to yet another victim. At which time you can feel safe logging on as your former self again. Who knows, you might even miss him. Nah.

Start Speaking Techie!

Okay, so you don't know how to hotwire a mother board or replace an Ethernet card. That's all right. Everyone has to start somewhere. And the nice

> "In view of all the deadly computer viruses that have been spreading lately, Weekend Update would like to remind you: when you link up to ANOTHER computer, you're linking up to every computer that THAT computer has ever linked up to."
>
> —Dennis Miller

NOT SO BUDDY LIST: SIMONE'S STORY

Talk about being "buddy burned!" Consider the tale of "Simone," if you will. Simone met a guy at a nightclub, but played it cool and didn't go home with him that first night together. Instead, the two sweaty dancers promised to meet the next morning, a Sunday, at a quiet little coffee shop halfway between both of their apartments.

When he actually showed up, looking twice as refreshed and rested as she felt, the two of them sat and shared a few cups of coffee and a biscotti or two as new age music twinkled angelically in the background. People came and went but Simone and her coffee buddy, we'll call him Joe (get it?), just shot the breeze and soaked up the warm, rich aroma of their quiet little coffee bar together.

When the noon hour came, Simone announced that she was going to church and Joe looked duly impressed. He'd heard a lot of blow-offs in his day, but going to church was a new one. To not make the morning a total loss, he lightheartedly suggested they exchange phone numbers.

Simone, still playing it cool, suggested they exchange e-mail addresses instead. Joe smiled and jotted his down on the back of a coffee stained

coaster. Simone reciprocated and the two parted ways amicably enough.

Later that same evening, while Simone was online tinkering with her Web page and getting prices on a weekend trip she'd been looking forward to for months, Joe's e-mail address popped up in the corner of her screen.

Though she hadn't quite gotten around to adding Joe to her buddy list just yet, his e-mail nom de plume was simple enough to remember: Joe22@samurai.net. It sat there glowing a bright, bold blue in its little buddy box next to his simple message "Hello?" as she tried to read the flight information on the screen hidden behind it.

Another ding later his name glared in its little box and this time the "HELLO?" was insistent, written in all caps. Why, that was practically the Internet equivalent of shouting!

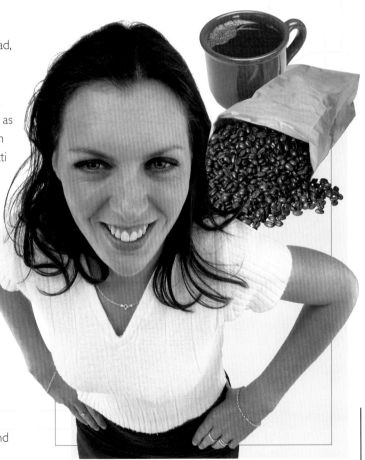

Not knowing what to do, Simone keyed in a similar greeting at the bottom of the box and hit "send," seeing her message pop up in the box just below his name. Obviously, still hopped up on caffeine from earlier that afternoon, Joe22 had been busy typing in her e-mail address and adding it to his buddy list.

She smiled to think he thought her important enough to add to such a personal list, and then moved on to her travel plans. But out of the corner of her eye, she kept looking for that glowing blue Joe22 address to keep popping up.

She didn't have to wait long. Joe22 was obviously just online cruising around, not doing much of anything, and seemed to have plenty of time on his busy little hands.

"Still there?" asked Joe22 as she tried to work.

"Hello out there?" he typed.

"Simone?" he clicked. "Still out there?"

Every time she tried to answer him, another blue Joe22 message blinked at the top left-hand corner of her screen and beat her to the punch. She considered herself a decent typist, but this guy was a regular rabbit! Just as she was finishing typing her first message in reply to his first *six*, Joe22 popped up again. "Fine," he keyed in rather churlishly. "I guess you've got better things to do than answer me. I'll try again tomorrow."

Simone chuckled that she could have such a pouting effect so quickly. It usually took her several dates to have the same impact on her other boyfriends. But then, she had to remind herself, this was no boyfriend, this was a "buddy."

The next day at work she thought about her new buddy often. She pictured his gentle hands as they had clasped his oversized coffee cup in the shop during their almost three hours together the previous Sunday morning.

She tried, with hindsight, to spot clues to his cyber-outburst of the night before. He'd seemed funny, gentle, and sweet, not only at the coffee shop, but also at the club. A lot of guys she'd dated wouldn't even have shown up the next morning, especially if she hadn't gone home with them the night before.

In a way, she thought, his little buddy-list blow up was sort of cute. Maybe he liked her after all. Soon, however, work interfered and thoughts of her new buddy were crowded out of her head. Later in the afternoon she received an "urgent" project, (weren't they all?) that would require her to work online that evening at home.

Later, with a half-eaten microwave dinner propped

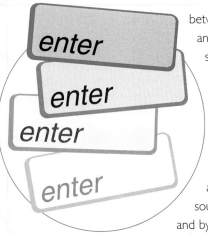

between her keyboard and her mouse pad, she surfed the net for help with her project, which was due the next morning. Before she knew it, Joe22 was at it again. Dings sounded left and right and by the time she'd finished running two search engines and printing out several documents for her project, there were no less than *eight* Joe22s littering a crowded buddy list box in the back corner of her computer screen!

Joe22: "Hello, hello, hello?"

Joe22: "Simone, you there?"

Joe22: "Hey, buddy, you around?"

Joe22: "I know you're there, you can't hide. I put you on my buddy list, you know, and it says you're online. AOL wouldn't lie to me now, would they?"

Joe22: "Humph. Fine. AOL wouldn't lie, but maybe *you* did when you said you'd be my buddy."

Joe22: "Fine, you don't want to talk to me? WHY DID YOU GIVE ME YOUR STUPID E-MAIL ADDRESS?"

Joe22: "Hey, Simone. Forget it. I'm taking you off this buddy list forever. It's called a list because there's more than one person on it, you know. Can your stupid Simone head grasp that concept? TWO people, not just me sitting here clicking away and waiting for a response that's never to come."

Joe22: "Why, why, WHY did I ever add you to my buddy list in the first place? I should have known that whole coffee shop deal was a blow off in the first place? Why did I show up? I'm such a loser. LOSER. Nope, no. Stop that, Joe. My shrink told me not to place the blame on myself anymore. It's your fault, YOUR fault you little—"

There was more, but by then Simone had logged off. Project be damned, she'd set the alarm for 2 a.m. and log back on then. Her Internet connection would be quicker anyway, and hopefully Joe22 would be long gone. Her fingers were shaking as she set the alarm clock and retired to bed, having been "buddy burned" for the first time.

It was a long time getting to sleep that night, and her last thought before she finally drifted off was: "Damn, I really liked that little coffee shop, too."

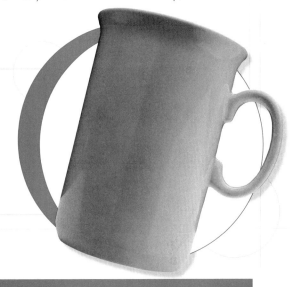

A MATCH MADE IN CYBERSPACE

The Internet is turning into the "Mother of all Matchmakers." According to a new study conducted by the Fortino Group, 66 percent of future marriages between members of "Generation Y" will originate from chat room romances. The survey also reveals Generation Y—kids who are now ten to seventeen years old—will spend almost one-third of their lives logged on to the Internet, which amounts to about twenty-three years. By comparison, the typical Gen Xer will only spend around ten years of his or her life online, while Baby Boomers will only spend about five and one-half years glued to the computer screen.

TECHNO TANGO

With financial (not to mention technological) success, one would hope, comes romance. (Otherwise, what's the point?) And now that the geeks and geekettes of yesterday are the studs and studettes of today, savvy techno-twosomes are suddenly worrying more about what they're wearing underneath all of those cool cyber clothes.

After all, those underwear from summer camp that still have your initials on the waistband in permanent marker aren't exactly a torrid turn-on! But then, neither are your Apple logo panties or IBM monogrammed boxer shorts.

No, it's quite a heady trip, suddenly becoming a cyber sex symbol. You must now dress according to your silicone station in life. For it's one thing to toil away in your darkened computer lab every night, munching on cold lo mein and not caring whether it stains your drab BVDs or Fruit-of-the-Looms.

Yet it's quite another to suddenly be the rage of the dot.com office, with your fat stock options and bulging 401(k) plan making the hotties in marketing swoon with digital desire.

Let's face it, your Hyper-Text Markup Language (not to mention your loins) are in high demand these days. It simply won't do to run around wearing the same old underwear day after day like you did when you were a geek, a nerd, or a bookworm. After all, geeks, nerds, and bookworms are suddenly "hot" partnership properties, quickly replacing male models, quarterbacks, and rap stars as today's most eligible bachelors.

So what's a poor guy to do when he's so busy depositing all of those hi-tech stock dividend checks he can't slow down long enough to shop for a decent pair of underwear? Double-click to find out:

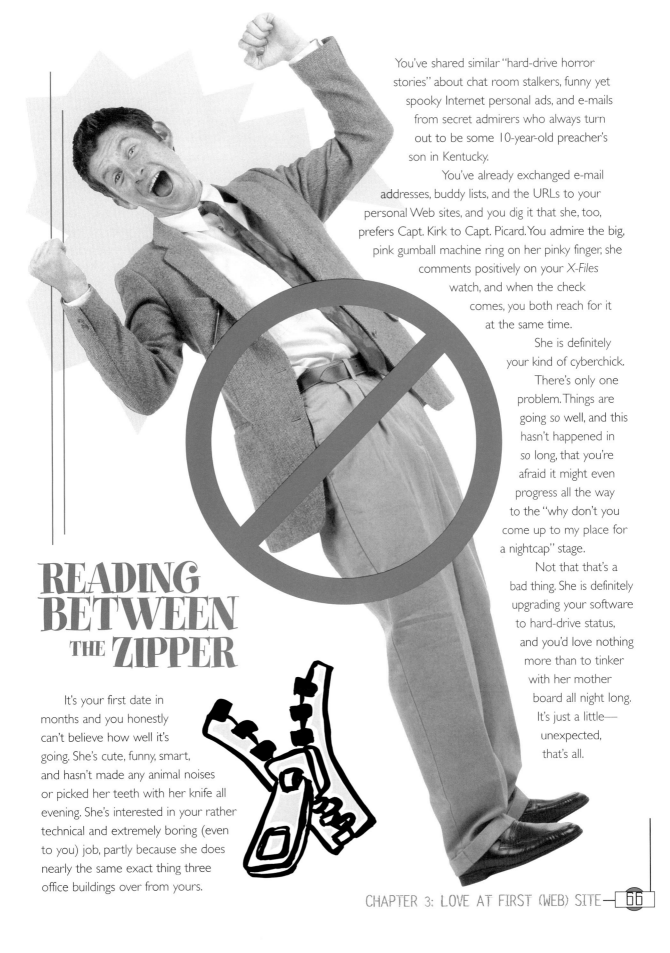

You've shared similar "hard-drive horror stories" about chat room stalkers, funny yet spooky Internet personal ads, and e-mails from secret admirers who always turn out to be some 10-year-old preacher's son in Kentucky.

You've already exchanged e-mail addresses, buddy lists, and the URLs to your personal Web sites, and you dig it that she, too, prefers Capt. Kirk to Capt. Picard. You admire the big, pink gumball machine ring on her pinky finger; she comments positively on your *X-Files* watch, and when the check comes, you both reach for it at the same time.

She is definitely your kind of cyberchick. There's only one problem. Things are going *so* well, and this hasn't happened in so long, that you're afraid it might even progress all the way to the "why don't you come up to my place for a nightcap" stage.

Not that that's a bad thing. She is definitely upgrading your software to hard-drive status, and you'd love nothing more than to tinker with her mother board all night long. It's just a little— unexpected, that's all.

READING BETWEEN THE ZIPPER

It's your first date in months and you honestly can't believe how well it's going. She's cute, funny, smart, and hasn't made any animal noises or picked her teeth with her knife all evening. She's interested in your rather technical and extremely boring (even to you) job, partly because she does nearly the same exact thing three office buildings over from yours.

Your last twenty-seven dates have terminated long before dessert and, expecting much the same to happen tonight, you'd paid little attention to your undergarment of choice, never for a single nanosecond believing that anyone but you and your cat, Data, would ever actually see it.

In fact, so heedless were you, you can't even remember which carefully segregated underwear drawer your current pair came from: action adventure or sci-fi? Why, oh why didn't you wear your lucky bikini briefs like the guys in your local chapter of the *Spawn* fan club suggested?

Sure, she might have thought you were a little too in touch with your feminine side had she seen them, but better that than to think you're a little too in touch with your alien side.

"Calm down, calm down," you tell yourself silently as you settle the bill and she delicately handles the tip. "Nothing will probably even happen anyway. Quit flattering yourself."

"So listen," she coos, toying suggestively with the after-dinner mints she's so carefully arranged into miniature green genitalia on the tablecloth, "why don't you come up to my place for a nightcap?"

"S-s-sure," you stammer, a last minute inspiration solving any and all undergarment uncertainty. "Let me just use the restroom first."

You can zip into the men's room, spread out luxuriously in the handicap stall, shed your Darth Vader, Mulder, Hercules, or Robocop skivvies, slip back into your relaxed-fit, date night cargo pants, and go "au naturel." She might think you a little crude, but she certainly won't be able to crack any jokes about your inner child.

Who knows, it may even turn her on.

"That's okay," she says, diffusing your plan, not to mention your fantasy, instantly. "You can go at my place. It's right around the corner."

Sweating bullets in the driver's seat, you park, ride the elevator up to her charming place, and then bolt for the bathroom. But she surprises you with a keyboard-strengthened grip and pulls you back into an amorous embrace, quickly sending any and all intergalactic paranoia out of your underwear-addled brain.

Five seconds after her minty breath has made mincemeat of your ears, you barely even hear your zipper being tinkered with. Five seconds after that, however, her stinging laughter reminds you of what you'd been dreading for the past fifteen minutes.

"Great," you sigh, standing there in the middle of her living room with your favorite pants around your ankles and your favorite Interterrestrial Alien doing little to hide your sudden enthusiasm at your fortunate turn of events.

"I'm sorry," you apologize, grasping at straws. "They

were a gag gift from my little brother and I haven't done my laundry lately and—"

Cut short in your ramblings by the sound of yet another zipper, your daring date strips off her tiny chinos to reveal a furry creature of her own.

"Wow," you say, "I didn't know they made Big Bird panties!"

"Oh, yes," she purrs, introducing *Sesame Street's* lovable lovebird to outer space's hairiest hero on an up close and personal basis. "You'd be surprised what you can find if you just look hard enough."

"Would I?" you query, surprised that you can actually be so witty when your mind is 3,000,000 light years off in a galaxy far, far away.

"Why don't you try looking," she quips, Big Bird's tail feathers bouncing gingerly as she pads away into the darkened bedroom, "... and find out for yourself. After all, are you a man—or a monster?"

You answer her loud and clear: "Growl!"

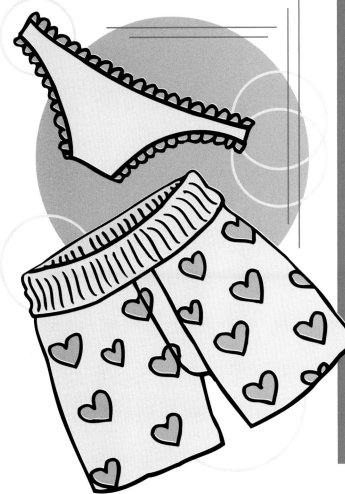

COMMONLY USED INTERNET ACRONYMS
(To be used for World Wide Wooing!)

AFK	**Away From Keyboard**
PDA	**Public Display of Affection**
BRB	**Be Right Back**
BTDT	**Been There, Done That**
BTSOOM	**Beats The SH*T Out Of Me**
BTW	**By The Way**
RTFM	**Read The F**king Manual**
FAQ	**Frequently Asked Questions**
FOFL	**Falling On Floor Laughing**
FWIW	**For What It's Worth**
PITA	**Pain In The Arse**
GAL	**Get A Life**
GG	**Gotta Go**
HAND	**Have A Nice Day**
HTH	**Hope This Helps**
HTML	**Hyper-Text Markup Language**
IRL	**In Real Life**
LMAO	**Laughing My Ass Off**

CYBERSLEUTHS & CYBERSTALKERS

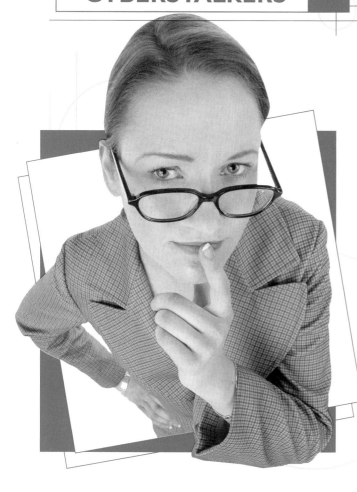

Despite the Internet's tremendous influence on our daily lives, many modern singles have come to see cyberspace as just one more place to be rejected, humiliated, confused, and let-down. Let's face it, we can't all be Tom Hanks and Meg Ryan and meet fellow movie stars each time that slightly annoying techno-voice announces, "You've got mail!"

In fact, for some, this seemingly innocent message has become a literal harbinger of doom. Consider the following story of a thoroughly modern techno-woman, we'll call her "Felicia," and her just as technically proficient cyberstalker, whom we'll call "Philip."

Felicia was tired of the usual dating scene, and decided, like many modern women, that, if she could find sweaters, books, and CDs online, why not find a

boyfriend as well. Felicia, being smarter than the average cybergal, decided to skip the cheesy chat rooms and even the supposedly secure online personal ads. She didn't even subscribe to an online dating service with a cute name like "Boyz 'n Bytes" or "Log on for Love!"

Instead, Felicia became a cybersleuth. A digital detective hunting for that most elusive of all suspects: love. She spent every waking minute looking for "clean" Web sites and "safe" places to hang her heart. She ran searches for teachers and preachers. Engineers and train engine collectors. Boy Scout leaders and Little League coaches.

From Web sites across the country, for little more than the price of her Internet provider and a few extra eye drops each night, she downloaded pictures of middle-aged men in baseball caps, publicity stills, soccer shin pads, and Elks Club group photos.

She gathered clues from personal Web sites across the country. Who was getting divorced? Who already had kids? Who'd been arrested and for what? Armed with plenty of information and even more e-mail addresses, she approached several of the most likely candidates. Yet, surprisingly, few were impressed by her determination and desire, and even fewer responded.

"Has someone out there already tried this route?" she asked herself as her time online dwindled considerably. "Is *that* why people go to chat rooms and read personal ads?"

Then, on a whim late one night, her eyes strained, her neck crooked, her back sore, she typed the word "kids" into her search engine and sat back and waited. She didn't know what made her do it, but she thought that maybe a man who liked kids and geared a Web page toward them couldn't be all bad.

In moments she came back with hundreds of hits, bordering on the thousands, really, yet only one with any real potential: a single man who wrote poetry for children and had a Web page listing everything about himself but his waist size. Which, judging from the full color glamour shot gracing his site (looking very artsy in his tweed jacket while holding his latest children's book and sitting on a slide), wasn't all that big.

She enjoyed his poems, and even quoted her favorite one to all of her friends the next day at work:

KING OF THE BACKYARD

By Philip the Poet

His frogs leapt off.
His horsefly flew.
His goldfish turned
Three shades of blue.

There used to be
Three fuzzy geese.
But they flew south
And broke their lease.

An ostrich once
Patrolled the grounds.
But then took off
In leaps and bounds.

He walked outside
To feed his swan,
But found instead
An empty lawn.

"I've no pets left,"
The boy exclaimed.
But then looked down
A tad ashamed.

For there sat Leo,
His final boarder:
A lion with...
An eating disorder!

"What the heck?" she thought. "Why not?" She clicked on Philip the Poet's e-mail address and, as 2 a.m. crept into 3, composed a short note pointing out their shared love of children's poetry, small waists, and classic children's toys.

After all, a guy who still wore

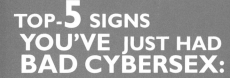

tweed and wrote for kids couldn't be all that bad, right?

The next day after work she poured herself some coffee and checked her e-mail. Lo and behold, there was one from Philip.

"Dear Fellow Lover of Children's Poems," the lengthy e-mail read, her pulse racing despite the fact that she had yet to take a sip of coffee. "I enjoyed your e-mail very much. It was nice to get a message from an adult for a change, especially one of the female persuasion. It gives me a chance to share with you some of my adult poetry. Would you like to hear some? Good. Here goes: There once was a man from Nantucket…"

While Felicia read on, surprised, no, shocked at the number of words that rhymed with "penis," she made a quick mental note to check into those chat rooms and personal ads after all.

None of them, she realized, could be quite as wicked and nasty as one kids' poet who'd gone very, very bad.

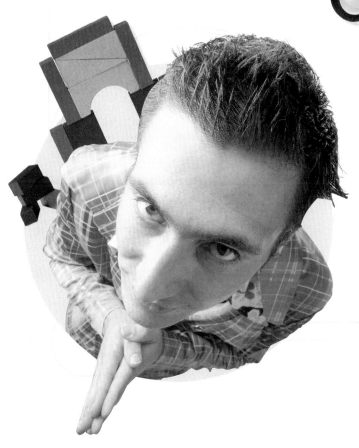

TOP-5 SIGNS YOU'VE JUST HAD BAD CYBERSEX:

5 An e-book version of the *Kama Sutra* suddenly appears on your desktop.

4 That's funny, the models in your Victoria's Secret screensaver weren't giggling before…

3 You start to get mysterious e-mail alerts from Viagra.com.

2 You're pretty sure that wasn't *really* Tom Cruise.

1 Your computer has to "restart" itself.

4
NIGHT LIFE, OR: CLUELESS WITH A COCKTAIL

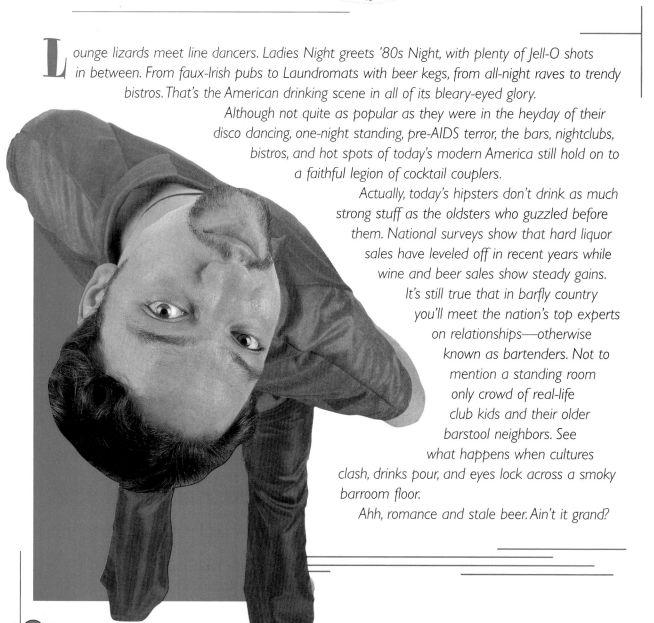

ounge lizards meet line dancers. Ladies Night greets '80s Night, with plenty of Jell-O shots in between. From faux-Irish pubs to Laundromats with beer kegs, from all-night raves to trendy bistros. That's the American drinking scene in all of its bleary-eyed glory.

Although not quite as popular as they were in the heyday of their disco dancing, one-night standing, pre-AIDS terror, the bars, nightclubs, bistros, and hot spots of today's modern America still hold on to a faithful legion of cocktail couplers.

Actually, today's hipsters don't drink as much strong stuff as the oldsters who guzzled before them. National surveys show that hard liquor sales have leveled off in recent years while wine and beer sales show steady gains.

It's still true that in barfly country you'll meet the nation's top experts on relationships—otherwise known as bartenders. Not to mention a standing room only crowd of real-life club kids and their older barstool neighbors. See what happens when cultures clash, drinks pour, and eyes lock across a smoky barroom floor.

Ahh, romance and stale beer. Ain't it grand?

BAR HOPPING

Choosing a bar is a lot like choosing an apartment: you want to feel safe but comfortable, cozy but with plenty of room to roam around in, and you'd prefer a clean bathroom. Accordingly, today's bars are catering to their clientele more than ever before.

From hot appetizers to cozy booths, from domestic microbrews to imported tequila, the days of the corner dive are rapidly fading away like so much beer foam on your cocktail napkin.

Surely, with all of these new themed bars, from Irish to Hollywood, sushi to coffee, your chances of finding Mr. or Miss Right inside are bound to improve as well. Right? The answer is yes, if you take as much time to choose the bar you're going to frequent as you do the lounge lizard or trophy babe you're going to pick up inside. After all,

every bar is not only unique for its hanging kilts or life-size Arnold Schwarzenegger statues, but for its individual clientele as well.

Therefore, we'd like to kick off this round of selections on cocktail coupling with a brief introduction to all of those different kinds of bars out there, not to mention the different drinkers, and daters, inside. So raise your glass, and keep on reading.

BE A SPORT

Ahh, the thrill of a packed sports bar. The roar of the crowd. The pitching. The spitting. The scratching. The striking out. The fresh smack of leather on skin. The slide into home plate. Hey, what the—they have TVs here, too?

After all, today's sports bars are far from being "males only" establishments. If they were, would the drink special of the day be a banana daiquiri? Naturally, the very idea of a sports bar as a dating hot spot has as many pros and cons as a

A GUIDE TO HIDDEN DRINK MEANINGS

If your date orders:

- Pabst Blue Ribbon
- Mai Tai in a souvenir glass
- Scotch on the rocks
- Sex on the Beach
- Piña Colada
- Shots of tequila
- Dirty martini
- Banana daiquiri
- Six diet sodas
- The nightly drink special

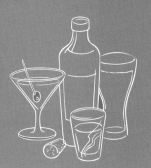

It means:

- he's a cheap date.
- she's a virgin.
- you'll be driving home.
- she's a tease.
- he'll appreciate your edible panties.
- he'll need Viagra after last call.
- she's secretly kinky.
- she'll go "ape" for your Tarzan yell.
- he's hoping you'll pass out.
- she has a crush on the bartender.

bookie's clientele. For starters, don't complain if you go home with a jock, ladies. After all, you knew what you were getting into when you walked inside. Or did you think those referee stripes on the bartenders and cocktail waitresses were zebra skin instead?

Guys, you too. Don't be shocked if the little cutie you end up taking home likes to call the shots in the bedroom. (This is a bad thing?) After all, didn't you spot her slaughtering the rest of the boys at the electronic basketball game? You knew she was going to be a tomboy going into the relationship. You just didn't seem to mind at the time. (Hmm, could that be because she challenged you to that beer bong race?)

All in all, sports bars could quite possibly be the most honest pick-up joints on the face of the earth. After all, most of them are brightly lit, no one's asking the barkeep to change any of the forty-two TV screens to A & E, and everyone's there to see somebody "score." Now, whether it's you or the local hockey team is another matter.

THE LUCK OF THE IRISH

One pleasant side effect of faux-Irish pubs is their faux-clientele. After all, the decision to come to an Irish pub over say, a disco or a bistro, is an entirely conscious one. A statement, if you will. A *bold* statement that goes something like this: "I'm tired of the usual bar scene. And I'm tired of the usual bar babes or bar buds. I want something different. Something new. Something… exotic. But someplace where I can still speak the language. Hey, what better place than Ireland?"

Therefore, most of the people you'll find in the local Shamrock Sam's or O'Reilly's Tavern are just trying to add a little spice to their lives. Accordingly, to succeed in a place like Finnegans or McCourts, your attitude should determine your altitude. *You* must be that little hottie in the corner's exotic exchange

student. Or that hunk on the barstool at the end's "spice of life." Hey, and if you can throw in a fake Irish accent, you'll be right at home.

It doesn't hurt that many Irish pubs, for some strange reason known only to their proprietors, are located in hotel lobbies. Naturally, this makes the opportunity for one-night stands a no-brainer, considering a good three-fourths of the bar's patrons need only to stumble up a few flights of stairs and make sure their room key still works to fall into bed. Follow them upstairs, and you'll find *more* than a pot of gold!

Shaken, Not Stirred

Another popular trend in bars these days are the martini/cigar bars popping up on every yuppie street corner known to man. Thanks to the hit movie *Swingers* and the success of *Cigar Aficionado* magazine, martinis and cigars are suddenly all the rage.

Naturally, you can expect a rather large poser potential inside any of these trendy establishments. Which is fine, as long as your approach fits in. For instance, it's always a good idea to bone up on *The Wall Street Journal* or at least the Business section of your local paper before strolling into the local gin joint. For some reason, the same people who are spending thirteen dollars on a glass of gin and olives and fourteen dollars on a so-called "good" cigar also claim to be savvy business people.

Naturally, a well-rounded portfolio, no matter how factual, is as good a pick-up line as any.

On the other hand, if everyone else in the room is wearing Armani and Chanel, you might not want to saunter in wearing your tie-dye tank top and cargo pants. Then again, maybe that's *just* the outfit to wear. Nothing's more attractive than a tidal pool of originality in a sea of sensible sameness. Of course, it might cost you a pretty penny waiting around for that tight-ass at the end of the bar to discover the inner you, but if you've got enough left on your credit card to make it to last call, we say go for it! (Just remember the Visine.)

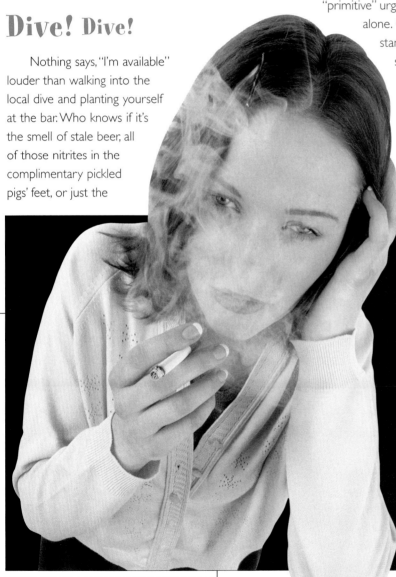

HANGOVER Helpers

Everything but the Kitchen Sink!

If you can locate the blender (nope, that's the toaster) pour in one can of V-8 (minus the can), a banana (minus the peel), and two aspirin. Throw in an egg, a little lemon and lime, then blend until smooth (or as smooth as possible). Consume in one gulp. (Or at least one sitting!)

Dive! Dive!

Nothing says, "I'm available" louder than walking into the local dive and planting yourself at the bar. Who knows if it's the smell of stale beer, all of those nitrites in the complimentary pickled pigs' feet, or just the clinging smell of desperation hanging in the room, but dives are a great place to go when you're feeling those "primitive" urges. And the nice thing is, you won't be alone. Chances are, you'll probably find a standing room only crowd of likeminded sorts swilling their two-for-one draft beers and watered down margaritas as they chain smoke cigarette after cigarette, all the better to form that sexy (i.e. husky) voice just in time for that last call proposition.

Dives are honest, straightforward, and affordable. Sure, they're getting beaten down or bought up by all of the themed bars and chain establishments cropping up on every interstate, intersection, and side road in the country, but there's still enough around to come in handy in a pinch.

Another nice thing about dives is their 24-7 mentality. Since they're usually open all day, every day, you're not restrained to just showing up on Friday or Saturday night when it's "happening." Every night is Friday night in a dive, and every hour is happy hour.

Say you feel the loneliness creeping up your loins at nine o' clock on a Tuesday night. Do you sit around watching the Discovery Channel for relief until 6 p.m. on

Friday? Heck no. That's what dives are for. Run on down, buy the desperate little cutie sitting next to you a drink, listen to her sob story, tell her yours, and then check your watch. Chances are, she'll have work tomorrow also. All the more reason to pop the question that much sooner.

Try that maneuver in some hoity-toity martini bar, mister!

Chain, Chain, Chain!

Finally, we close with the exact opposite of the dive bar, the chain bar. You know the chain bars. They're all over the place. You can't step out to pick up a carton of milk or buy a gallon of gas without passing three or four of them on your way. It's amazing we're not all alcoholics! You'll recognize them by their potentially perky names: Bennigans, T.G.I. Friday's, Chili's, Tony Roma's, Jungle Jim's, Houlihan's, etc.

Pick one. It doesn't really matter. They've all got the same clean-cut wait staff, the same twelve-pound menus, and the same generic memorabilia hanging from the dusty rafters: sleds, fishing poles, antique Coca-Cola signs, and rusty skates. You know the drill.

Surprisingly, despite their extremely high cheesiness factor, chain bars can be a great place to meet the girl or guy of your dreams. (Or, at least, your daydreams.) For one thing, they're extremely popular, which naturally shoots up your odds for picking up a member of the opposite sex. For another, they're reasonably priced, which means you can hang there for longer, thereby further increasing your odds. They're also loud, which helps if you're a noisy breather or have the hiccups. They're generally well lit, which helps avoid those nasty, "Hey, I didn't see that hump on your back" scenes in the harsh light of morning. And above all, if you strike

out in one, chances are you can walk three paces next door and find a whole other crop of chain bar clientele to try those smooth moves on. (Or practice some new ones.)

Probably the best thing about chain bars, however, is the assumed safety factor involved. After all, it's Bennigans, only normal people go there, right? It's not like some creep is gonna hit on me. Sure, lady. All the creeps hang out at Planet Hollywood. You're safe at Chili's.

Sure you are.

THE BARTENDER'S GUIDE TO RUM AND ROMANCE

Tending bar may not be the "oldest profession in the world," but it must surely run a close second. After all, it's a pretty tight race between "wine" and "begat" for the coveted "word that appears most in the Bible" award. Surely the respected profession of bartending wasn't far behind wine's inebriated invention.

And if bartenders are by nature experts in the art of "mixology," they must all certainly minor in the mysterious world of "dateology." After all, while most bar patrons are too sauced by the end of the night to properly research this long lost art, bartenders are still on the clock and wired from all that free coffee and soda. Therefore, they see and hear *everything*.

Naturally, they could write a book on all of the misfired come-ons,

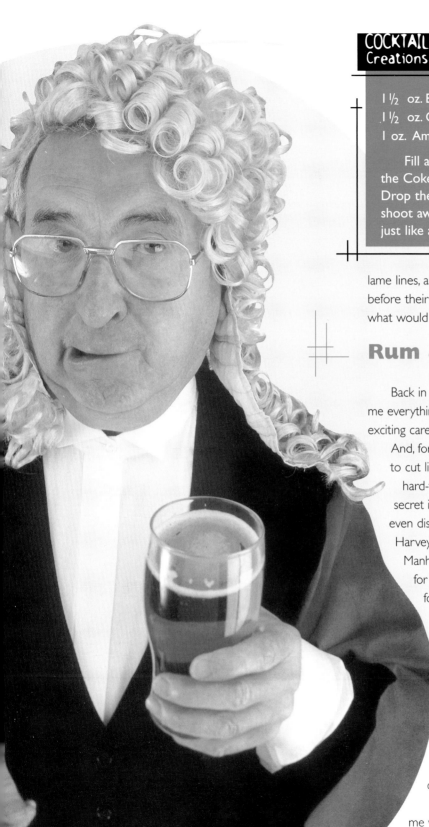

COCKTAIL Creations

Dr Pepper

1 ½ oz. Beer
1 ½ oz. Coca-Cola
1 oz. Amaretto

Fill an eight-ounce glass with the beer and the Coke. Then fill a shot glass with Amaretto. Drop the shot glass into the larger glass and shoot away. If you drink it fast enough, it tastes just like a Dr Pepper!

lame lines, and far-fetched flirtatiousness that passes before their all-too-jaded eyes night after night. Yet what would such a book contain:

Rum & Romance 101

Back in Bartending School, they said they'd teach me everything I needed to know for, in their words, "an exciting career in the growth industry of mixology." And, for the most part, they did. I learned how to cut limes just so and even how to open up those hard-to-handle cocktail umbrellas. I learned the secret ingredients for a great margarita mix and even discovered the mystery behind the coveted Harvey Wallbanger. I learned how to mix Manhattans for the senior citizens, cosmopolitans for all the Sarah Jessica Parker wannabes, daiquiris for the tourists, and even those silly, pseudo-sexual shooter drinks for the college crowd.

They even taught us the "real" secret to bubbly bartender banter: subscribe to the local newspaper! This simple and inexpensive trick taught me to read the sports page for small talk, the horoscopes for wisdom, the business page for stock quotes, and the funny pages for those quick one-liners my customers love so much.

But the one thing they didn't teach me was how to be what all bar patrons secretly, and some not-so-secretly, hope for in a really great bartender: a matchmaker.

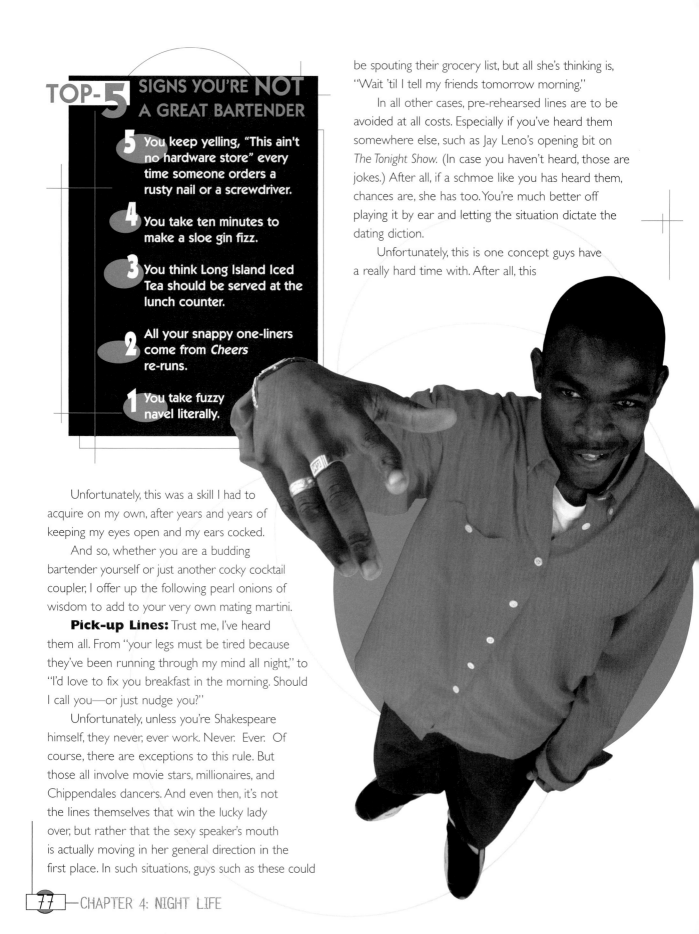

TOP-5 SIGNS YOU'RE NOT A GREAT BARTENDER

5 You keep yelling, "This ain't no hardware store" every time someone orders a rusty nail or a screwdriver.

4 You take ten minutes to make a sloe gin fizz.

3 You think Long Island Iced Tea should be served at the lunch counter.

2 All your snappy one-liners come from *Cheers* re-runs.

1 You take fuzzy navel literally.

be spouting their grocery list, but all she's thinking is, "Wait 'til I tell my friends tomorrow morning."

In all other cases, pre-rehearsed lines are to be avoided at all costs. Especially if you've heard them somewhere else, such as Jay Leno's opening bit on *The Tonight Show*. (In case you haven't heard, those are jokes.) After all, if a schmoe like you has heard them, chances are, she has too. You're much better off playing it by ear and letting the situation dictate the dating diction.

Unfortunately, this is one concept guys have a really hard time with. After all, this

Unfortunately, this was a skill I had to acquire on my own, after years and years of keeping my eyes open and my ears cocked.

And so, whether you are a budding bartender yourself or just another cocky cocktail coupler, I offer up the following pearl onions of wisdom to add to your very own mating martini.

Pick-up Lines: Trust me, I've heard them all. From "your legs must be tired because they've been running through my mind all night," to "I'd love to fix you breakfast in the morning. Should I call you—or just nudge you?"

Unfortunately, unless you're Shakespeare himself, they never, ever work. Never. Ever. Of course, there are exceptions to this rule. But those all involve movie stars, millionaires, and Chippendales dancers. And even then, it's not the lines themselves that win the lucky lady over, but rather that the sexy speaker's mouth is actually moving in her general direction in the first place. In such situations, guys such as these could tactic involves active listening, as opposed to just nodding your head and popping off with an occasional, "You are so right."

My advice is to skip the lines altogether. In fact, as a rule, guys should avoid speaking as much as possible in a bar. Especially as the night goes on. Not only does this give the impression that they are listening, but it goes a long way toward cutting down those awkward "open mouth, insert foot" moments they tend to find themselves in so often.

Flirting: This is a lost art that, in *my* opinion, has no chance of getting resurrected anytime soon—in this century or any other. Most guys' idea of flirting is to not steal money from her pocketbook until she's really wasted.

On the other hand, guys who do consider themselves "good" at flirting often go way, way overboard with the attention they slather on: Standing up every time the girl even squirms in her barstool, let alone gets up to use the powder room or buy a pack of smokes. Lighting her cigarette before it's even out of the pack. Snapping at the waitress for a refill every time his intended victim even thinks about taking a sip of her drink.

The girls are just as guilty of over-flirting as the boys, however. Most women in bars consider crossing their legs, licking their lips, and flipping their hair flirting. Luckily, most guys do too.

Picking up the Tab: Thanks to the sexual revolution and so-called "equality in the workplace," this timely tactic is now safe for both sexes. However, the messages sent are often very different.

For instance, if a guy buys a girl a drink, it's not exactly a subtle message. He's basically saying, "Look, I think you're cute. Cute enough, in fact, to spend money on. Naturally, this money is an investment of the short-term variety—as in, how many drinks will it take to get you drunk enough to go to bed with me?" Naturally, unless the girl's been living under a rock her entire life, she reads this message loud and clear.

Girls, on the other hand, rarely buy drinks for anyone else except other girls. This is one of the last few bastions of the fairer sex. They're stuck with menstruation, pregnancy, labor, and hot flashes; it's only fair that they should get a few free drinks along the way.

Of course, when a girl does buy a drink for a guy, the message is loud and clear: "Stick around. I've got plans for you."

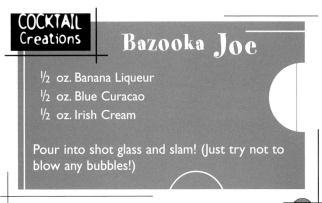

COCKTAIL Creations

Bazooka Joe

½ oz. Banana Liqueur
½ oz. Blue Curacao
½ oz. Irish Cream

Pour into shot glass and slam! (Just try not to blow any bubbles!)

Lighting Her/His Cigarette:

This is a classic, no-nonsense pickup ploy. It works for both sexes, costs little more than a gas-station lighter or, if you're really cheap, a pack of free matches from the bar, and is just subtly aggressive enough to get your potential partner's attention.

Unfortunately, it's just a little too generic these days to be very effective. After all, everybody does it. And everybody knows it. So nobody takes it seriously. It's a little bit like movie violence. After a while, you just get desensitized.

Naturally, as one who's consumed enough second-hand smoke on his job to fill three lungs with cancer, my suggestion is to skip the whole smoking bit altogether. Sure, it's a little phallic. Yes, it's pseudo-sexual. But so is a lollipop.

Eye Signals:

Bars tend to be a tad noisy, whether they offer live music or not. So eye signals are extremely important in the fine art of flirting. Unfortunately, most boozy bar patrons consider winking and staring to be the only acceptable form of eye signal. Such extreme eye behavior, naturally, leads to lots of 911 calls by the bartender. Girls report rampant "winkers" to the local ER for fear that they're suffering from a seizure or epileptic fit, and the "starers" just get reported to the police as spooky stalkers. Either way,

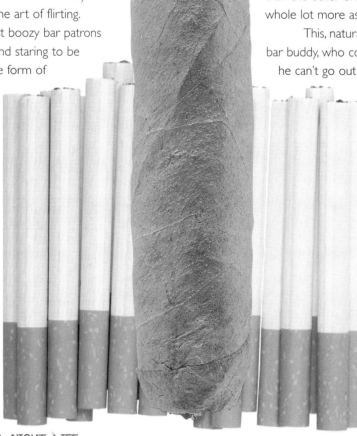

neither tactic attains the desired results.

The Buddy System:

This is a rather sneaky tactic employed by members of both sexes quite equally. Not to mention liberally. Once again, each sex employs such desperate measures for different reasons.

Guys tend to go to bars with a buddy for one reason and one reason only: to avoid looking like the single, desperate lounge lizards they are. Of course, friendly conversation and a little male camaraderie never hurt anybody, even of the male persuasion. But for that, both guys could have simply ordered a pizza and a six-pack, and watched ESPN back home.

But as bar buddies, they get to play it cool and make it seem as if neither of them is there to pick up chicks, which, naturally, is a lie. In all honesty, they both are. But in my experience, bar buddies don't last very long. Invariably, one bar buddy is better looking than the other one, and ends up scoring a whole lot more as a result.

This, naturally, upsets the "butt-ugly" bar buddy, who comes up with excuses why he can't go out with the "buff" bar buddy. In which case the buff buddy finds another butt-ugly buddy to bar hop with and repeats the cycle all over. Eventually, when he runs out of butt-ugly buddies, he simply shows up unattached and keeps looking at his watch anxiously, exclaiming to any and all that he can't imagine what's keeping his "buddy" from showing up. Either tactic usually works—for the buff buddy anyway.

Girls are another matter. Girl buddies are used more for protection than penetration. Girl buddies are a life raft in case of potentially disastrous situations. These include the "stud who turns into a dud," the "cute guy who's just escaped from the local mental hospital," and the "sweet talker who turns into a stalker."

While few of these are life-threatening, none is pleasant and all require the swift extraction that a female bar buddy can provide.

Naturally, the smoky world of rum-soaked romance is full of ever-evolving tactics—kind of like the next popular vodka. And, as long as the beer foam and olive juice don't smudge the ink in my little black bartender's guide, I'll be able to bring them to you as they evolve.

But hey, while we're waiting, how about a drink?

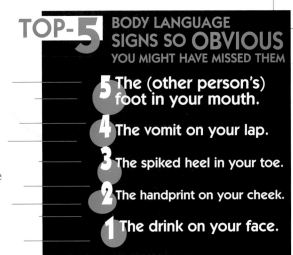

BODY LANGUAGE FOR THE COCKTAIL CLUELESS

Well, here you are again. Another Saturday night and no date. And, like the many countless, endless, mind-numbing, interminable nights before this one, you shower, shave, and splash on a little cologne and head down to the local watering hole in search of a little "action." Yeah, right.

If tonight is indeed like all the rest, you'll go home broken-hearted and empty-handed. Unless, that is, you stop by for that late-night order of Nachos Bell Grande you usually pick up at the Taco Bell across from your apartment complex.

Ah, but tonight won't be like all the rest. No broken heart. No empty hands. No nachos. No mild sauce. You're just sure of it. And, to back you up, you have the curled up, dog-eared copy of *Boning Up On Body Language* you've been reading all week.

After all, knowledge is key. And with this particular key, you intend to unlock the ancient secrets of body language that have heretofore been a well-guarded

"secret" language to you.

Naturally, since you decided to spend the last remaining moments of "happy hour" in the front seat of your Honda Accord cramming for tonight's festivities by reading the book's introduction for the twelfth time, the bar is packed by the time you go inside.

But no matter. With your newfound understanding of the language of the body, you stride confidently to the bar and proudly order one of those snazzy new microbrews you've heard so much about. (After all, wasn't one of the book's chapters called, "Actions Speak Louder Than Words!"?)

Naturally, you sip it contentedly from a safe distance in between the jukebox and pool table as you study your quarry for the evening. After all, you don't want to rush things. Unfortunately, that wiry brunette leaning against the foosball table keeps distracting you.

Of course, that could be because she's got legs for miles and a smile to match. Not to mention flowing hair, flawless skin, and a hard body. Still, this *is* a popular bar with the hotties. And you've ogled your share of young women before.

But there's something special about this girl's body. Could it be her body is actually "speaking" to you? After all, her legs are crossed at the ankles as she stands there sipping her margarita seductively.

Doesn't that "mean" something? Surely it must. In fact, you seem to recall a chapter in your book called, "Feet: Windows to the Silent Speaker's Soul." It had

Sex in the Parking Lot

½ oz. Chambord Liqueur
½ oz. Vodka
½ oz. Apple Schnapps

Blend the ingredients, shake with ice, and strain into a large shot glass. For city-folk, this is a variation of the more famous (but less realistic) "Sex on the Beach."

mentioned something about women crossing their legs and what it meant.

Yes, yes. It's all coming back to you now. Crossed legs were definitely a sign that a woman was interested. But was she interested in *you*? That was the real question. Heck, was she even interested in anything at all. After all, she wasn't actually crossing her "legs." Her ankles were crossed. Is she interested?

What exactly did your book say about that? Naturally, you can't whip it out and start examining it for clues. Although, that big plastic stand currently holding the bar's nightly drink specials could probably cover it. No, no, she'd definitely lose interest if she glanced over and spotted you sticking your head in a book. This was a bar after all.

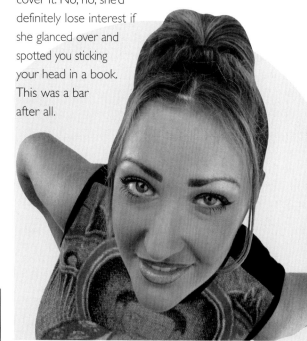

Okay, the crossed ankles aren't sending any signals. Look for something else. Let's see. Hmmm. Whoa? Was it you or did she just toss her head back. You didn't exactly need a body language book to define that hidden message. Crossed ankles *and* a head toss? She might as well be asking for your phone number!

Unless . . . well, what if a fly just flew past her ear? What if she was having some kind of seizure? What if she had Tourrette's syndrome and was getting ready to spew obscenities any second? Okay, okay—focus. Man, if you could only consult your handy book.

All right, wait—did she or did she not just wink at you? Oh man, oh man. Could it be? Did she really wink at you? Why, there was a whole chapter devoted to the one-eyed wink. No mystery there, but—what if—it was less of a wink and more of a tic? After all, she was a beauty, no doubt, but are you the kind of beautiful person (on the inside) who could spend the rest of your life with a woman who blinked constantly? As in, non-stop?

Okay wait, now she's twisting her hair. You had that one down cold. Right? If a girl twists her hair around a finger while talking to you (or, in this case, while standing within six feet of you), it most certainly denotes interest in what you are saying, how you look, hold yourself, dress, etc.

Really?

What if it just means she's got ants in her pants and needs something to keep her hands busy? What if it means she's interested in the guy behind you and is hoping her annoying habit of continually twisting that one lock of hair around her bony finger will eventually drive you away so she can show off some real body language to the fellow she's really interested in? What if she's just bored?

Oh, why, why did this all have to be so hard? As a guy, of course, your body language is much easier to read. If your eyes are open, you're interested. If your head is up off the bar, you're interested. Scratching yourself? Interested. Yawning? Still interested. Most likely she could pass you on the street three months later and you'd still be interested, a fact she could easily read by the way your forehead crinkles as she walks by. Why couldn't human foreheads be like those

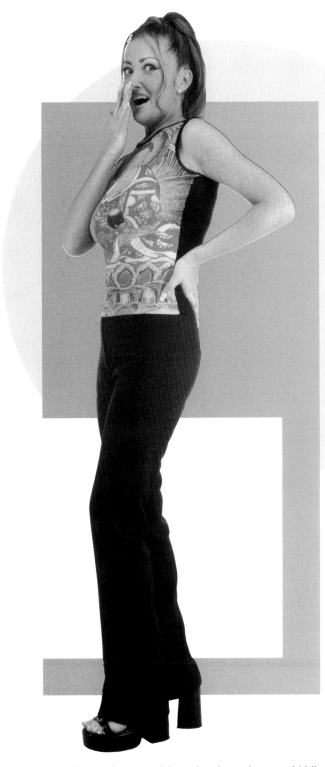

Then again, what good was knowing what someone might or might not be thinking about you if the rest of the barriers were still up? The approach. The come on. The flirting. The eye contact. The dance. The phone number. It would be nice if we could all agree on a separate sign for each of the above situations, a combination between sign- and body-language that would be internationally recognized and accepted worldwide. A universal language everyone could understand. But maybe everyone else *did* understand.

"But I already have signs for each of the above," you say? Great. Super. Good for you. Is it working? Does the girl across from you know that tapping your feet means the relationship is going too slow and that, instead of yet another drink, your little, tapping feet would prefer to dash across the street and get a hotel room? It's doubtful. More than likely, your prospect for the evening is assuming, "Wow, this guy must have a bladder the size of a peanut. I wonder if the rest of his equipment is similarly proportional?"

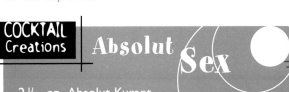

Eventually you leave not knowing what someone's body might have said to you. The girl at the foosball game drifted over to the pool table to talk to another guy. And that was that. Oh, well, at least you bought the book on sale. That means there's probably enough change in your pocket for that order of nachos on the way home.

proverbial stock quote tickers they have down on Wall Street? With a running commentary on what the forehead owner was really thinking? As in, "Yes, I'd like another drink with you." Or, "No, you creep, just get away from me before I call the cops!"

COCKTAIL Creations — Absolut *Sex*

2 ½ oz. Absolut Kurant
1 oz. melon liqueur
2 parts cranberry juice
2 parts 7-Up

Mix it up and drink it down. Just make sure to mix it well. After all, you don't want to suffer from premature intoxication! (Or do you?)

LADIES NIGHT, OR: LEAPIN' LOUNGE LIZARDS

SHE SAID

So you've finally decided to try out Ladies Night, huh? It's gotten that bad? Or don't you get enough sexual harassment at work? Maybe you just haven't managed to get your yearly quota of lounge lizards yet.

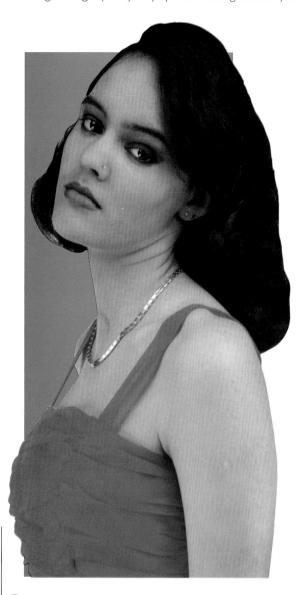

No matter, you have your reasons, and that's all that matters. Of course it is.

So, let's see. What's the scenario? It's a weeknight, that's a given. No self-respecting bar owner in his right mind holds a Ladies Night on the weekend. After all, his bar's sure to be packed already. Right? So is it a Tuesday? Or a Wednesday?

Hmm, most likely it's a Thursday. That's the perfect night for Ladies Night. The working women are completely stressed by now and only have one last morning to look forward to going into work. Why not be hungover? And the college gals have had it with exams, lab fees, and Must-See TV.

Okay, so it's Thursday then. Now, whom are you going with? Well, you're obviously not showing up stag! Are you? If you're that desperate, you might as well just slip into a pair of fishnet stockings and ten-inch heels and flash a little thigh down in the red light district. So, chances are you and a couple of the other single gals down at the office, hair salon, or department store have buddied up and decided on a "girls night out."

Okay, fine. Now, what are you wearing? Not the little sequin number again. Honey, it's Ladies Night, not "Lady Impersonator's Night." Try not to look so . . . desperate. Let's go with the black cocktail dress, simple pearls, heels but not *heels*, and leave the fishnet stockings at home.

All right, re-do the bangs one more time, lick your lips, toss some Tic-Tacs in your backpack purse, and hit the road. Now, who's driving? You haven't thought of that? Well, you better start thinking about it. Unless, that is, you want to get stuck downtown when Sheila, your "easy" friend from accounting, suddenly decides that she wants to turn Ladies Night into Gentleman's Morning with whatever sleazeball catches her eye at last call.

And don't *you* drive! For heaven's sake. Not unless you look forward to taxiing three big-haired gals around town at 1 a.m. trying to dissuade them from suppressed shopping sprees at every adult bookstore on the way home. Make up some excuse why you have to meet them there, silly.

That way, if it's lame you're out of there after one or two rumrunners and a bowl full of beer nuts. On the other hand, if a bus full of unattached, recent med school (or modeling school) graduates pulls up looking for Ms. Right, you'll at least be available.

Now that that's settled, all that's left is to pick the club. What are you in the mood for? Naturally, your choices here are a little bit limited. Most of the classier joints shy away from such blatant customer come-ons as Ladies Night. So that little bistro in the hip part of town you've been dying to try is probably out of the question. As are all of the other places you'd normally frequent if you were actually thinking straight at the moment.

Nonetheless, a quick review of the Lifestyles section of your local paper lets you know that you're not entirely out of luck. There's that '80s club, 8-Traxx. Dancing, discount drinks, and desperate dudes? It doesn't get much better than that. But wait: Donnie's Disco Dome has some killer drink specials just for the ladies. And Happy Harry's boasts, "ALL Ladies Drink FREE 'til midnight!" Which, you hope, is well past your girlfriends' curfew.

So, after a quick consensus, you and the girls plan to meet at 8-Traxx at nine. (After all, meeting at eight would've been just *too* cute.) Besides, that's just enough time to swing home and get gussied up and grab a bite to eat, but not quite time enough to settle in on the couch getting hypnotized by the latest sitcom that's about to get cancelled.

Naturally, you get there a little early because you want to scope the place out first just to make sure it isn't on the wrong side of town, crowded with rowdy Hells Angels, or just another secret location favored by the mob for dumping bodies. Plus, you have no intention of going inside alone. Remember?

Finally, you see a familiar face as Harriet from Sales pulls up in that flashy sports car she's leasing and still can't really afford. She's followed shortly by Jenny in IT,

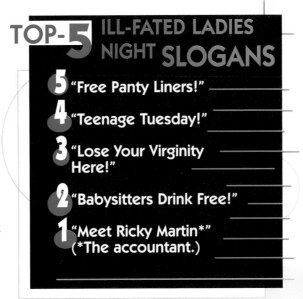

TOP-5 ILL-FATED LADIES NIGHT SLOGANS

5 "Free Panty Liners!"

4 "Teenage Tuesday!"

3 "Lose Your Virginity Here!"

2 "Babysitters Drink Free!"

1 "Meet Ricky Martin*" (*The accountant.)

Mona from Marketing, and finally the easiest of the bunch, Sheila, pulls up. And, now that the gang's all here, in you go.

Since the cover charge is nixed on this, *your* night, and your drinks are free ('til midnight, anyway), this leaves you "free" to mingle. Of course, since you came with all the friends you have in the world, you cling together like four geeks at a junior high school dance and cluster desperately at the bar. There, squeezed in between several other packs of wary women just like yourselves, you make endless small talk about your boss and complain ceaselessly about that pervert from the home office.

"Work is the curse of the drinking class."

– Oscar Wilde

As you eye the competition surreptitiously around the lipstick-smeared straw of your second Tom Collins, you realize that the term Ladies Night is taken quite literally at 8-Traxx. Why, besides the two bored bartenders, the bloated bouncer, and that creepy manager in the zoot suit up in the DJ booth, the estrogen dew point in the noisy club is hovering at about, oh, 100%!

Still, it's better than a frozen dinner and a bad video back at your place, so you decide to lighten up and enjoy your friends and put your dreams of Mr. Right away for yet another night. But then, at around eleven, just as you and the girls are tiring of the "Oh, man, remember *this* song?" routine every time they play a Donna Summer tune, an amazing and unexpected event occurs.

Men show up. One or two at first. Then a slow trickle. And then, as if that proverbial buff busload had just pulled up, you turn your head to silently signal the DJ *not* to play "I Will Survive" for the forty-second time and see that the testosterone level now exceeds that of the estrogen by at least a good 4:1!

Naturally, these are not the hard-bodied M.D.s you'd dreamt of meeting. In fact, the closest these guys will ever get to being a doctor is when they eventually pass out from cologne poisoning and are rushed to the ER. Still, it's refreshing to hear a masculine voice order a beer for a change.

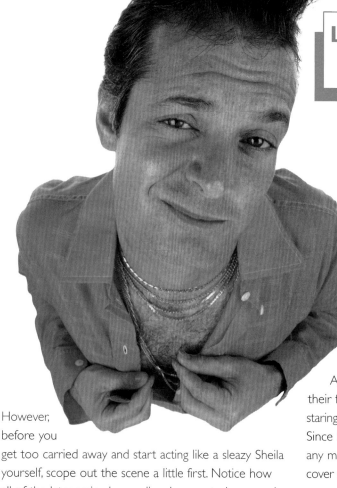

However, before you get too carried away and start acting like a sleazy Sheila yourself, scope out the scene a little first. Notice how all of the latecoming lounge lizards seem to know each other, not to mention the bartenders, bouncer, and even the DJ, by name.

Witness how each one stakes out his territory with practiced precision, either sidling up to an unsuspecting gaggle of girls immediately, or playing it

cool and waiting a few sips or two first. Sniff the overpowering scent of over-the-counter, Brut splash-on cologne. Feel the heady mixture of polyester and velour slide along next to you as the hairy dude inside of each orders yet another Bud longneck.

Then ask yourself: Is it really worth it?

And when you answer yourself, gather your girlfriends together and hit the road. Immediately. After all, there's always that guy from the home office to chat up tomorrow.

He's sort of cute. Sort of.

LADIES NIGHT: TAKE TWO 2

HE SAID

Yes! Finally, it's Ladies Night. The night I've been waiting for all week long. Now, let's see. Is everything in order? My cheesy pick-up lines have been rehearsed in front of a mirror? Check. Plenty of singles in my wallet to make it look like I'm a player? Check. Breath mints? Check. Too much cologne? Check. Four shirt-buttons undone? Check. Roll of quarters positioned just so in my tight silk slacks? Check *and* double-check.

All right, then. It's 11:01 p.m. The ladies have had their fill of free drinks and bad music. They've been staring at each other for a couple of hours getting antsy. Since it's Thursday, they still have work tomorrow and if any magic's gonna happen, it's gonna happen soon. The cover charge just went down for guys, the drink specials are over, I've got a wad full of dollar bills, and, away we go!

Here you go, Mr. Bouncer sir, there's three bucks for you. Now, how are the ladies looking tonight? Great? Super? Out of sight? All right, then. In I go.

Man, he wasn't kidding. Check out all that hair. Smell that cheap perfume. Look at the length of those legs. Nice rack! Now, let's see, if I can just squeeze into the bar here and get myself a drink. Wait. What's this? An unescorted female standing next to me. On ladies night? Imagine that.

"Can I buy you a drink, little lady?" I ask, trying to keep my focus above the neckline for a change. (Tends to avoid getting slapped.) A shy nod and the bartender hands over a beer for me, another Sea Breeze for my lady friend.

"So," I schmooze, glad I practiced all those pick-up lines in the mirror last night. "The heavens must be missing an angel 'cause I just found my star. Hey, wait. Where are you going?"

Shoot, I knew I'd screw that one up. Heavens. Angel. Star. Too many damn words. I should have just stuck with a good, old-fashioned grunt. It ain't exactly original, but it's pretty darn hard to screw up.

Wait, hold your horses. There's another fine filly standing across the room looking lonely and bored. And I'm just the man to light up her life. Now, let's see what she's drinking. Hmm, looks like another one of those damn Sea Breezes to me. What are these girls, all in cahoots? Here, let me finish up my beer and, bartender, another round for me and my new lady friend. Thank you kindly.

All right, here we go. "Hi there, ma'am. I couldn't help but notice you standing here looking lonely and bored with a half-empty Sea Breeze in your hand. You wanna slam that one right quick and I'll hand you this fresh new one if you don't mind and, whoa, hey, you weren't kidding. Here's your fresh one and, wow, I've never seen a girl do that before.

"What, you want another one? Okay, fine. Hold your horses. Let me finish mine here, gulp, gulp, gulp. I'll just signal that fine little cocktail waitress and order us another round, thank you dear, and, here you are. Let's try sipping this one so we can talk a while."

"What's that? You don't speak English? Don't fret, darlin'. The language of love is universal. Hey, come back!"

Shoot, another one bites the dust. Boy, I should have had dinner tonight. All these beers are going straight to my head. Oh, well, that's all right. At this pace, I'm sure to find a lucky lady before my first trip to the little boy's room.

HANGOVER Helpers

(The Morning After) Ladies Night

Trick your battered brain into thinking it's getting a little "hair of the dog" with this Bloody Mary impostor: combine eight ounces of Bloody Mary mix, one jalapeño pepper, one garlic clove, three cubes of ice, and a shot or two of water in a blender. Blend until "chunk-less" and then consume.

Now, there's a looker. Tall. Strong-boned. Distinguished looking. And not too prissy the way some of these gals like to turn their noses up at a hardworking ladies man like myself. Let's see, what's she drinking? A beer? Now that's my kind of gal.

Here, let me finish this draft and bartender, two more of the same. Thanks a lot. Now, for the approach. So far, so good. She hasn't slapped me yet. Wow, and with the size of those hands, it looks like she's a fighter. All right, I'm setting her beer down, good, fine, now I'm sliding it over. Okay, she's nodding. Wait, was that a smile? Now she's sipping it, now she's draining it. All right, just like I thought. A girl after my own heart!

"I can resist everything except temptation."

– Oscar Wilde

Okay bartender, let's set 'em up again.

"Phew," I say, accepting our drinks and paying the bartender with a few of my dwindling singles. "I ran into you just in time. Any more rounds of drinks and I'm not so sure I could 'perform' later on, if you know what I mean."

The pretty lass with the hairy arms, strong hands, and muscular frame just nods and says, in that husky voice of hers, "I know exactly what you mean."

And, as we toss back beer for beer and chit and

chat about everything from baseball to hockey, hot rod engines to *Playboy* magazine, it sure seems that way. Glad I came to this ladies night. And just think, another round or two and this little lady, well, not so little actually, but this healthy hottie is gonna be helping me pass the evening in all sorts of new and unique ways, if you know what I mean.

Hey, is it just me, or is the room spinning? Phew, I'll have to take it easy on those beers. What's that? It's last call already. All right, well, I've still got a few bucks left. Why not? My partner sure seems willing, let's toss 'em back before they kick us out of here.

"Wow," I say, attempting to stand and being helped by my brand new lady friend. "Thanks a lot. Hey, you didn't look so tall sitting on that barstool for the last two hours. Well, what'll it be honey? Should I call you in the morning, or just nudge you?"

"Look, pal," she says, escorting me out to the nearly empty parking lot. "Thanks for the drinks and all, but, I'm not so sure you'd want to take me home with you."

"Nonsense," I grunt, admiring her muscular legs and ample bosom. "I want to take you home in more ways than one, if you know what I mean."

"Yeah, listen," she says, her voice a little more than just husky now. "I know exactly what you mean. After all, I let you buy me all those drinks back there, the least I can do is be honest with you. I'm not really a girl. I'm a guy. I'm just a little down on my luck and so I dress up like a lady for the free drinks. You're not mad, are you?"

"Heck, yeah I'm mad," I'd like to say. But at the moment I'm busy getting rid of all those great draft beers, the hard way. When I'm through, Mrs. Mister notices that the roll of quarters in my pocket has shifted a little and doesn't look quite as flattering anymore.

"Hmm," he says, climbing onto his Harley Davidson and firing her up. "Looks like I'm not the only impersonator in town."

As I watch her, ehhr, *him* drive away, I have just one thing to say: so much for "ladies" night!

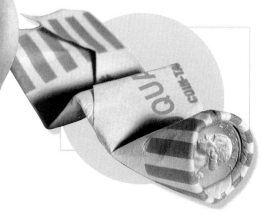

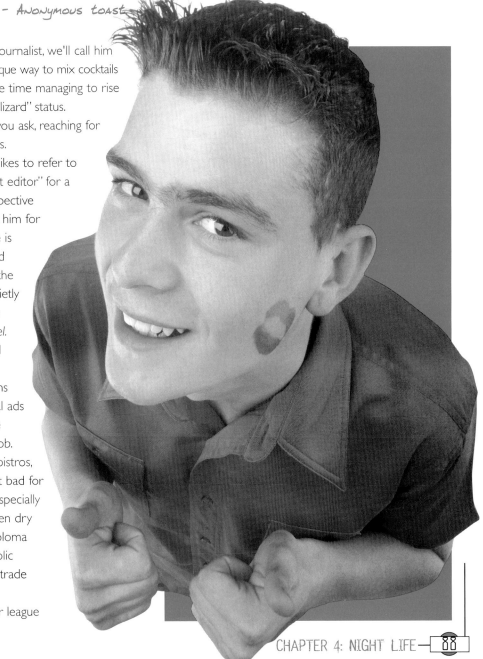

MAX AND MINDY: COCKTAIL COMPANIONS

*"Here's to you and here's to me,
I hope we never disagree.
But, if that should ever be,
To hell with you, here's to me!"*

— Anonymous toast

A certain professional journalist, we'll call him Max, has "hit on" a rather unique way to mix cocktails and dating while at the same time managing to rise above the dreaded "lounge lizard" status.

"How does he do it?" you ask, reaching for pen and paper to take notes.

Well, for one thing, he likes to refer to himself as an "entertainment editor" for a "big, local daily." When prospective employers or girlfriends ask him for a business card, however, he is conveniently always out. And when he says the name of the daily, it's always mumbled quietly and mixed in with a sudden coughing fit: *The Thrifty Nickel.*

Max may not be proud of the fact that his weekly "entertainment" column runs right alongside free personal ads for tractor parts and garage sales, but he does love his job. Reviewing local pubs, bars, bistros, and lounges each week isn't bad for a twenty-five-year old kid, especially considering the ink's not even dry on his Journalism school diploma yet. Why, older, more alcoholic veterans of the newspaper trade would kill for such a gig.

So, armed with a minor league expense account and a major league ego, Max and an always unnamed "companion," (read: "lucky lady of the week," or, if an off-week, "roommate who wants a couple of free beers") head out to check out the local bar scene. There's no note-pad involved. No fancy, hi-tech recording equipment, either. Just Max and his draft-beer addled brain a couple of hours after last call as he clicks away at his battered, coffee-stained laptop looking out of his apartment window at the deserted streets below.

Max loves his work, and it shows. Only the grungiest, most disgusting bars ever get a bad review and even those that do receive a framed copy to display right between the Slim Jims and the pickled pigs' feet behind the bar.

As a single guy, of course, Max's columns tend to fluctuate between the cozy couples' bars he frequents when he's dating someone, or the sleazy singles bars he reviews when his "companion" for the night is his roommate or the leftfielder from the *Thrifty Nickel* softball team.

As such, his 300 or so faithful readers have been treated to a cornucopia of local bars, ranging from biker hangouts to sterile, themed Irish pubs, from Laundromats with draft beer to French-inspired wine and cheese cafés.

Meanwhile, those same faithful readers have witnessed Max's love life rise and fall as well. For when his job is, after all, to go out and be sociable, it's hard to keep his feelings as close to the vest as say, a sports columnist.

Accordingly, Max's many and varied girlfriends have often made it to the first-name stage for his readers, (Usually just before she dumps him.) One girlfriend in particular, we'll call her Mindy, made it into Max's column a total of six times, a *Thrifty Nickel* record!

Readers were treated to the "blushing boyfriend" phase, as in Max's second column when he repeatedly referred to Mindy as his "beautiful companion" or "lovely companion," or, a first, his "longtime companion."

Eventually, readers learned

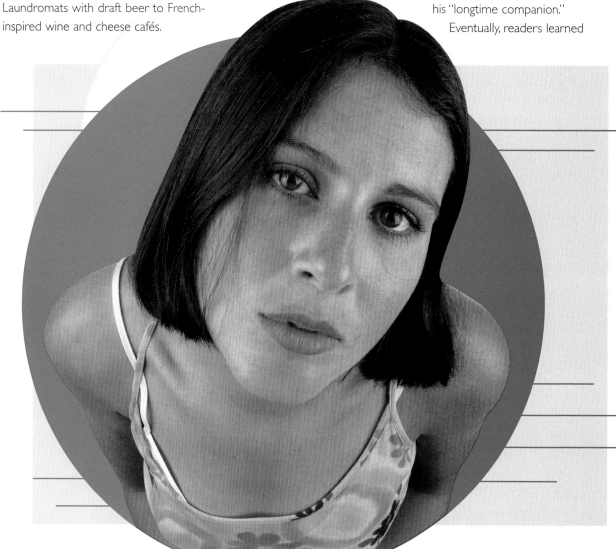

MINDY MAKES ME MAD!

Mindy's name, as Max quickly reeled her into his third column by titling it, "Mindy's Mad Martini," her favorite drink.

By his fourth column, readers knew Mindy was a bank teller at a local financial establishment, which later experienced a surprising surge in new accounts. Readers also learned that Mindy smoked Marlboro Lights. "But only when she drinks, folks," the wry columnist explained, waxing poetic, perhaps due to his current romantic bliss. And, of course, Mindy drank martinis. And lots of them, apparently, if one were to take Max's fifth column, "Mindy's Martini Madness," seriously, in which readers were warned that, due to Mindy putting such a dent in Max's meager expense account, there might not be a column next week.

There was a column, however, and it was to be Mindy's sixth and final appearance. Readers knew it would be a humdinger, too, as soon as they read the blunt title: "Mindy Makes Me Mad!"

Few readers would be able to remember the name of the bar reviewed in this blistering column, the first line of which read: "This reviewer respectfully wishes to apologize to his faithful readers, who, over the last six weeks, have had to put up with this naïve fool as he followed a martini-swilling, chain-smoking bank teller who made me diss my friends, not to mention my faithful fans, you: the readers. And I apologize again, in advance, if this last and final 'Mindy' column reads more like a raving rant and less like a bar review."

Max and Mindy, it would seem, were over, especially since Max's equivalent to a "Dear Mindy" letter appeared in black and white on 7-11 and Circle K newsstands all over their small town. Max went back to reviewing the local bars, pubs, and taverns, and Mindy transferred banks.

Max's readers remained faithful, of course, but couldn't help feeling a little misty-eyed upon reading Max's first Mindy-less column the very next week, as he and his old college roommate made the rounds that first sad and Mindy-less night.

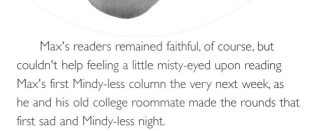

HANGOVER Helpers

Chicken!

If you're feeling gun shy of consuming yet another "drink" the morning after another big night of boozing, warm up a can of chicken broth and pour it into a bowl. Next "medicate it" with five shots of Tabasco and one egg for a cure that's sure to leave you feeling better. (Whether you can keep it down long enough to work is up to you!)

5
CINEMA COURTSHIP, OR: SEDUCTION FOR THE LAZY & BORED

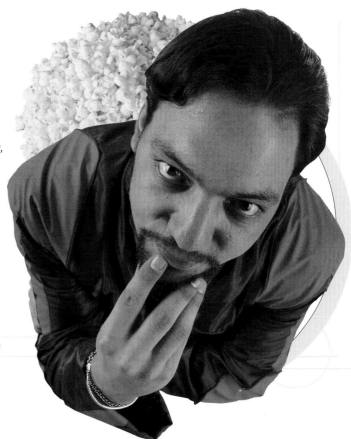

"**D**inner and a movie." It's the unfinished phrase with the implied ending, "and a night in the sack together." What movies can bring to relationships (or subtract from them) makes the cinema an integral part of almost any couples' (or potential couples'), uh, coupling (or uncoupling). Movies bring clever lines into play ("Say, nice beaver!") and serve as an early litmus test on how things might unfold in the future. ("Thank you, I just had it stuffed.") It teaches couples to give each other space: He's watching Die Hard 6 and she's watching Titanic, Frozen in Brine: The Adventure Continues.

Movies affect the posture men and women take with each other, not to mention the clothes they wear and even how they react. After all, who didn't wear a ripped sweatshirt and legwarmers after seeing Flashdance for the fifth time? (No, not you sir.) And who could forget ogling Sharon Stone cross and uncross her legs in Basic Instinct? (No, not you ma'am.)

And dating? Dating and movies go together like milk and cookies. Speaking of cookies,

remember the immortal words of Old Man Dunphy (Alec Baldwin) from Outside Providence, "Making sex is like a Chinese dinner: It ain't over 'til you both get your cookies."

DINNER & A MOVIE:
FREE ADMISSION TO THE **ULTIMATE** DATE

Dinner is one thing. Great. A little wine. Maybe some salad. The house vinaigrette? Sure, pour it on there. Rolls. Butter. Hmm, chicken or fish? Some pleasant conversation. Maybe even a little lighthearted flirting in between visits by the snooty waiter.

But, then what?

Movies? Yeah, they're good too. Super. Fine. Smell that freshly printed ticket to auditorium thirty-seven. Let the pleasant, bubbly bouquet of a ripe diet soda tickle your delicate nostrils. And popcorn? Where else can you get really good popcorn these days except at the movies?

> "You know **how** a **woman** gets a man **excited?** She **shows up**. That's **it**. We're **guys**, we're **easy**."
>
> —Quinn Harris (Harrison Ford) in, *Six Days, Seven Nights*

Besides, movies provide couples not only with a couple of hours of good old-fashioned entertainment, but they prime the conversational pump as well:

He said: "The symbolism of the condom in *Porky's Revenge* is simply too obvious to miss."

She said: "Indeed, but what about the metaphor of the opera in *Moonstruck*?"

Sparkling soda and sparkling conversation. Indeed. But, then what?

But, dinner and a movie—that's a date! But what is it about this coupling combination that has made it a true American ritual in the annals of dating history? Could it be those glamorous stars? Or is it that waiters and ushers dress alike? (Coincidence? We think not!) Could it be the prospect of eating twice in the same night? Or is it just the prospect of sharing two meaningful events with the same person?

While dinner and a movie can now be an intimate night at home, the two events grew up together as a way to get *out* of the house So, sit back. Smell that popcorn. (What, you don't have a microwave handy?) Put your feet up and enjoy the show. Don't worry, the admission's free!

ADMIT ONE

Sure, he didn't direct anything you can run down and rent from the local video store, but many Hollywood historians credit the Frenchman Louis Lumière as the inventor of the motion picture camera in 1895. Of course, most movie mentors date the true "birth" of the motion picture to D.W.

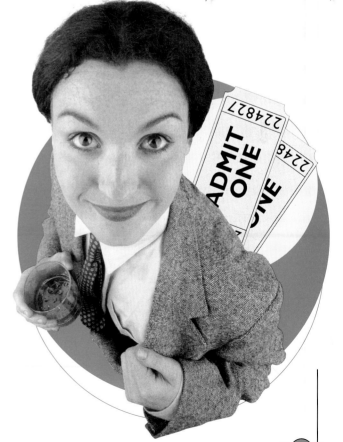

"Now that Billy tried to
mutilate her, do you think
Sydney would go out with me?"

—Randy (Jamie Kennedy)
in, *Scream*

Griffith's cinematic epic, *Birth of a Nation* in 1915.

And by as early as 1912, in a parallel universe,
lunch wagons in Providence, Rhode Island, had become
so numerous that they were actually blocking the city's
streets. Eventually a law was passed requiring them to
be out of traffic by 10:00 a.m. In order to keep serving
throughout the day, many wagon owners parked their
vehicles permanently in abandoned lots. Voilà! The
prehistoric Diner is finally born.

As the silent movie era progressed and cinema
courtiers grew by the hundreds, Wichita, Kansas was
about to make hamburger history as Walter Anderson
opened a diner prominently featuring hamburgers on
the menu. By 1921, he was in search of a business
partner to help him finance a fourth diner, so he joined

forces with Edgar "Billy" Ingram. They named their
enterprise White Castle.

Movies were silent until 1929, when a means of
recording sound that would actually match the moving
image was finally discovered. And, with the advent of
"talkies," another great restaurant chain was born.
Massachusetts. 1925. Howard Johnson, who owned a
small soda shop and newsstand in the town of
Wollaston, was asked to open a second shop in Cape
Cod. Unfortunately, he didn't have the funds. But he
persuaded a friend to open a restaurant using his
unique specifications and serving his successful products.
The idea worked so well that he continued to expand
his business in this way. By 1941, Johnson had an empire
of 150 franchises in the eastern United States.

First "talking pictures!" Then Howard Johnson's.
Could it get any better?

The answer, apparently, was yes. For studio heads
and movie stars, that is. After all, stars powered the
American studio system from 1934-1946. Various
studios, such as 20th-Century Fox, Paramount Pictures,
Metro-Goldwyn-Mayer, Columbia Pictures, and Warner
Brothers rose to power on the coattails of such
celluloid luminaries as: Clark Gable, Claudette Colbert,

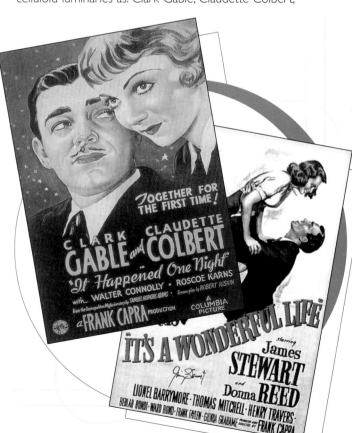

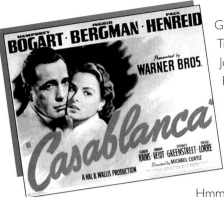

Gary Cooper, Spencer Tracy, Judy Garland, John Wayne, Henry Fonda, Jimmy Stewart, Cary Grant, Joan Fontaine, Humphrey Bogart, and Ingrid Bergman. Talk about star power.

Hmm, hearing all those names, not to mention watching them on the silver screen, must have made those fabulous flappers and hat-headed hunks hungry. Well, they were in luck. Some of the most famous restaurants in America opened during this Hollywood heyday, including The Rainbow Room at the top of the RCA Building at Rockefeller Center and the world-famous Trader Vic's. Movies hit a slight snag in the '50s, when the television set became a permanent fixture inside the American dream home. As a result, Hollywood tried everything from cinemascope, VistaVision, drive-in movies, and science-fiction films featuring bug-headed aliens as a desperate attempt to lure viewers back to theaters.

And, as if giant, radioactive, super-intelligent ants weren't enough to silence a courageous couple's rumbling stomachs, they had a whole new batch of appetite adventures to choose from. The soda fountain was a popular '50s fixture, offering the convenience of hopping from drug store to movie theater and back again for a true "dinner and a movie" home run. To top it off, "fast food" found its origins in the '50s when Ray Kroc bought out the McDonald brothers and offered cheap hamburgers, French fries, and milk shakes under their distinctive "golden arches."

While the '60s will be remembered for an impressive list of "meaningful" films, few of them stand out as truly great date movies. After all, most were gut-wrenching dramas or ground-breaking cinematic achievements. *Doctor Zhivago. In the Heat of the Night. The Graduate. To Sir, with Love. Easy Rider. 2001: A Space Odyssey. Bob & Carol & Ted & Alice. Midnight Cowboy.* Date movies? Hardly.

Dining in the '60s was another matter. Sure, the films were okay, but how about those restaurants? You've seen them. If the walls weren't covered with smiley faces, peace signs, and those big psychedelic flowers, then they were draped in gaudy blue wallpaper, gold frames, and macramé. Okay, they may have served a great veggie platter with soy milk on the side and those "funny" brownies for dessert, but who could withstand the nausea caused by the pea green Naugahyde chairs and nightmare orange shag carpet?

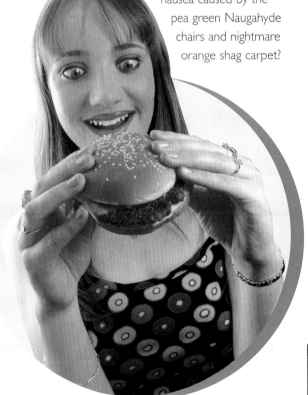

By the '70s, both movies and eat-in restaurants had been around long enough for the "dinner and a movie" date to truly have cemented itself in American culture. These were heady days for both types of connoisseurs. As for the movies, there was *The Godfather, American Graffiti, The Exorcist, Jaws, One Flew over the Cuckoo's Nest, Taxi Driver, Annie Hall*, and *Close Encounters of the Third Kind*.

As for restaurants, well, the prices weren't the only things being elevated. Social consciousness was being raised as well. In 1972, a group of friends who gathered regularly for collective meals in Ithaca, New York, decided to open the Moosewood Restaurant as a community project. In keeping with their political beliefs, it was a completely cooperative venture.

The food served was vegetarian, and the owners introduced dishes based on the cuisines of different countries. So, after waiting in line for hours to see *Star Wars*, you could grab a hummus pita and a little red zinger tea and pretend you were dining on Luke Skywalker's home planet.

Now, was there a better time for going on a classic "dinner and a movie" date than the roaring '80s? The movies, gems each and every one, kept coming and coming. And we kept going and going: *The Breakfast Club. Dirty Dancing. Pretty in Pink. Ferris Bueller's Day Off. Risky Business. Sixteen Candles. Weird Science. Top Gun*. The eyes truly water at the cinematic offerings of a bubble gum decade bent on nothing short of entertaining each and every one of us to death. Truly, those were the good old days.

Malls were the dating destination of the '80s, and with multiplexes cropping up at every shopping center from Minsk to Miami, the local mall was your all-in-one-

stop for movie and a dinner, both within a few feet of each other. Naturally, your choices were a tad limited. There were the inevitable, chain mega-munchie emporiums: Ruby Tuesday's, T. G. I. Friday's, and the odd Chili's or two. But other than that, the '80s still launched "dinner and a movie" to new heights.

The '90s were a confusing time for "dinner and a movie" daters. Sure, there were plenty of films to choose from. More than ever, in fact. But with the rise of independent films, was it still politically correct to go see a $200 million Bruce Willis spectacular when there, right next door in theater #49, was a sleeper of an independent gem from Australia about orphans, lab animals, and a one-legged prostitute? Somehow, however, we managed to muddle through a decade fraught with special effects and special moments. We cringed at *Goodfellas*. Sang "Hakuna Matata" to *The Lion King*. Wouldn't dare say *Candyman* more than twice. We got cozy at *The American President* and thrilled to such summer blockbusters as *Armageddon* and *Godzilla*. We cried at *Titanic*, and cried and cried and cried. And, then, of course, the best date movie of the decade, *The Blair Witch Project*, took us all by surprise just before the millennium.

Here was the perfect movie to cap off the '90s: an

independent film that was also a money-making blockbuster. We could be PC and entertained at the same time. (A new experience, to be sure.) Not to mention, there's nothing better than a good, old-fashioned scary movie to force those first, few hesitant hand-holding moments into sheer bear-hugging overdrive!

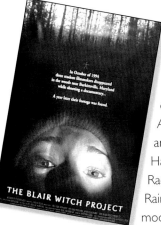

THE BLAIR WITCH PROJECT

The '90s also saw the rise of even more themed restaurants. And boy did they rise, and rise and rise and rise. Planet Hollywood. Hard Rock Café. House of Blues. Race Rock. Medieval Times. Rainforest Café. Depending on what mood you were in, you could ride electronic race cars holding a hot dog, take in a carrot malt shake for two, or eat with your fingers while watching two hacks joust with each other only a few feet away.

Of course, few know what the future holds for "dinner and a movie." Perhaps someone will invent a multiplex themed restaurant where you could sit and sop up Schwarzenegger salsa and chips while watching the Arnold himself cracking skulls and emptying bullets into innocent women and children.

Tums, anyone?

SAFETY IN NUMBERS: THE SUMMER BLOCKBUSTER!

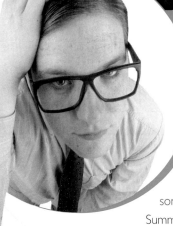

You can question whether taking a member of the opposite sex to a summer blockbuster can even be considered a date at all. For while it's one thing to sit cozily next to one another at a matinee showing of Charlie Sheen's latest straight-to-video bomb, enabling you to spread out arrogantly in a 400 person theater currently being occupied by you, your date, and a homeless man sleeping one off in the back row, a summer blockbuster is something else altogether. Summer movies are invariably overcrowded, and the stretch factor is usually slim to none. And when squeezed in between a family of eight on one side of you and a soccer team on the other, can either of you really say you've actually gone out on a date at all? After all, do you really feel comfortable

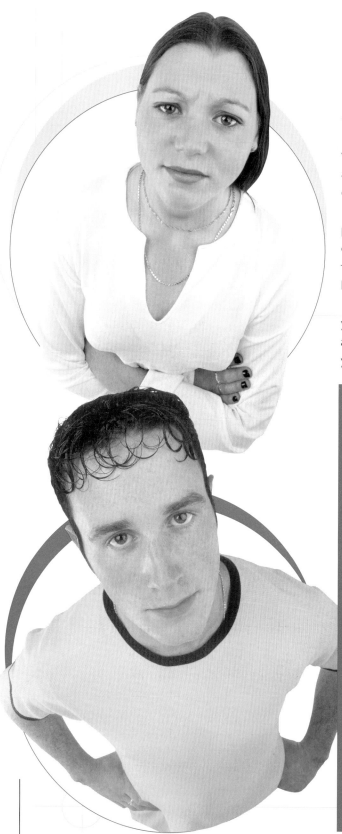

making out in front of kids, jealous couples, and senior citizens, all jammed into the theater like sardines in a can?

For another thing, today's cinematic blockbusters now rely heavily on overblown soundtracks and overdone special effects, both of which produce noise levels previously unimaginable. Accordingly, those once whispered "sweet nothings," are now shouted to one another as if from across a football arena, cutting down even more on the intimacy level.

On the other hand, a summer blockbuster is the perfect blind date, since the two of you can ignore each other for a full two hours before crashing back to reality for the long drive home (which might *seem* like two hours!).

Other dates to take to the summer blockbuster: your mother's friend's son, the podiatrist with the athlete's foot. That girl from work who's been hounding you to go out with her for years. Not to mention the

BASIC INSTINCT VOTED SEXIEST FILM OF ALL-TIME

Which film is the sexiest of all time? According to a survey by *US* magazine, *Basic Instinct* is the most erotic film of the last millennium while *Titanic* plays second fiddle, coming up just short of the #1 spot. Other facts from the survey:

● **20 percent admit they felt aroused while watching *Deep Throat*.**
● **47 percent think Tom Cruise and Nicole Kidman are the sexiest Hollywood couple, while 21% prefer Brad Pitt and Jennifer Aniston.**
● **20 percent think Will Smith and Jada Pinkett have a wild, wild time in the sack.**

one-night stand from last week who wants proof that he/she wasn't a one-night-stand after all, which one date at the movies should certainly prove without a doubt, especially since you'll never see him/her again.

For established couples, however, the summer blockbuster holds certain land mines and other "lethal weapons" of the verbal kind. Since these larger than life films are necessarily filled with larger than life stars, one must avoid getting too excited and spewing such relationship-stalling lines as, "Oh, you know me honey, I'm a big Sandra Bullock fan. I'd watch her in anything, or, out of anything, for that matter. What? Why are you looking at me that way? What'd I say?"

Other film-inspired "Fatal Attractions" include:

"Doesn't Mel Gibson have a great butt, honey? Honey? Where are you going?"

"You know why they call him the 'Italian Stallion,' don't you?"

"Remember when people used to tell you that you looked just like Sharon Stone, sweetheart? Boy, those were the good old days."

Jealousy isn't the only relationship trap set by the summer blockbusters, however. Any couple forced to stand in line longer than five minutes is headed for the inevitable "out in public, he/she is acting like an ass again" fight. Such "theater throw downs" can often ignite from a simple act like not buying enough popcorn, or buying too much, to not handing her ticket to the usher but instead letting her do it herself.

Other blockbuster battles include when you forget that he's lactose intolerant and ask for butter on the popcorn. Forgetting that she's allergic to Twizzlers and presenting her with a bag as a surprise. Calling him a moron when he spills your soda and you can hear it gushing down eight rows of chairs. Telling her it's her fault that you're sitting in the front row since she's the one who took so long getting ready when, after all, you can never tell the difference anyway.

Come to think of it, maybe couples who want to stay together should avoid the summer blockbuster altogether, while those "mercy dates" with nothing better to do should fill those long lines around the block instead.

BLOCKBUSTER vs. BARS: WHY CAN'T BOTH SERVE BEER?

Blockbuster and other pre-fab chain video stores have slowly been replacing bars in the minds of many young singles as a pick-up joint ever since they added microwave popcorn and soundtracks to their ever-expanding inventory.

For one thing, it's much easier to see a wedding ring under all of those bright, retail lights than it is buried three knuckles deep in the beer

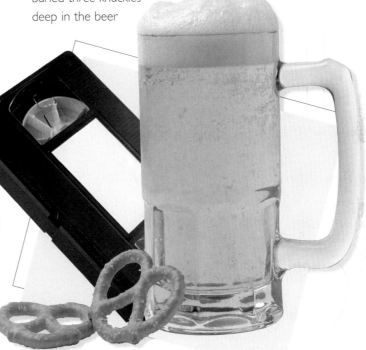

nuts down at the local tavern. And other visual clues to a potential suitor's marital or dating status are so much easier to pick up on as well:

The workaholic mother crouching down on power-suited knees for the latest *Teletubbies* extravaganza is obviously a sexual stop sign, as is the frustrated husband whining into his cell phone, "But we've already seen *The Horse Whisperer*." Such cryptic clues would have taken several hours, not to mention bar tabs, to glean in a dimly lit bar.

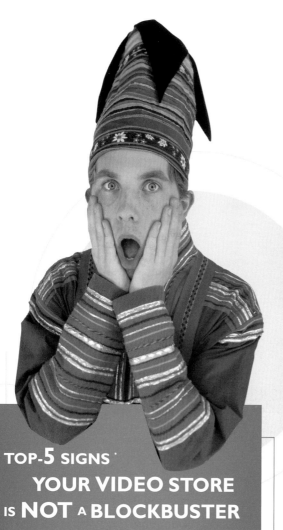

"**What's** the point of **sleeping** with you if it doesn't get your **attention?**"

— Carl Tippett (Lyle Lovett) in, *The Opposite of Sex*

Meanwhile, singles with an attitude show their hand just as clearly.

For instance, the Goth babe who's renting *Interview with the Vampire* for the twelfth time but whose eyes keep lingering over Adam Sandler's latest release is obviously prime for a Blockbuster night with any prepster brave enough to see past her black wardrobe, black lipstick, black eyeliner, black tattoos, and jet black hair. As is the hip-hop, Puff Daddy wannabe whose eyes keep lighting up every time he passes *Brian's Song*, which his teacher probably showed him in grade school. A passionate night of cuddling and fly boy fumbling is only a simple, nostalgic, "You know, I just rediscovered this great Run DMC album," away.

However, single shoppers aren't the only targets in video stores these days.

Even among those who consider themselves "attached," wandering up and down the endless aisles of vapid videos all alone is a sure sign that things are in trouble. (Or at least, *can* be with a little helpful prod from an observant ogler such as you.)

For instance, any guy who'd let his girlfriend fight the Friday night traffic and endless crowds alone, only to come home with a sappy stack of chick-flicks anyway, is a guy who's obviously just waiting until she falls asleep so he can sneak out and hit the local topless club for a little Boob Tube of his own.

Similarly, any woman worth her salt would never

TOP-5 SIGNS
YOUR VIDEO STORE
IS NOT A BLOCKBUSTER

5 Your late fee is whatever you can scrounge up in your car's ashtray.

4 *E. T.* is still in the "New Release" aisle.

3 *Schindler's List* is filed under "Comedy."

2 The only "candies" they sell are edible panties.

1 Your "membership card" is written on the back of a cocktail napkin.

"**You** know what the **twenties** are for? Having **sex** with all the **wrong** people. **Not** to get **married.**"

—Lilly Leonard (Bette Midler) in, *That Old Feeling*

trust her man to pick out the Saturday night video by himself. Unless, of course, she too is a huge fan of Jean-Claude Van Damme or Yasmine Bleeth. Here is a woman obviously willing (or eager) to lose her man to the belly-button-ringed co-ed who was two minutes late for the last Lilith Fair Live concert video still on the shelf. With one simple response to her innocent, "Now what am I gonna watch tonight?" the bemused boyfriend could quite possibly spend the evening consoling her in her dorm room with a *Poison Ivy* double feature.

> **"These** days, you have to **boil** somebody before you can **sleep** with them."
>
> —Paul Brenner (John Travolta) in,
> *The General's Daughter*

Meanwhile, the little woman back home is doomed to watch *Woman Scorned: The Betty Broderick Story* (again) on Lifetime until the half-hearted candles burn down and the take-out Chinese food cools.

DIRTY ON DVD: APHRODISIACS FOR THE EYES

There comes the point, of course, when movies fail to be the "safety net" of every new couple's dating landscape. When the mere crinkle of the movie section fails to bring the once-expected gleam to a partner's eyes. When popcorn can no longer be considered an appetizer and a Blockbuster night means that one of you is going to be sleeping on the couch.

Fortunately, this is no reason to eliminate movies from your dating diet altogether. After all, that's what the "adults only" section in your local video store is for. You know the one. Back there in the corner. By the free popcorn machine that's always mysteriously "out of order."

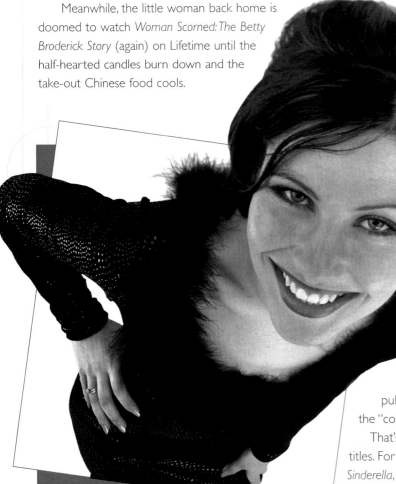

What's that you say? You've never been in there before. Well, why not? You're an adult, right? You can certainly vote and buy cigarettes and be drafted into the army. Why not find a few unexpected thrills right there in your local video store. After your old English teacher leaves, that is.

That's it. You're getting warm. Now put down that copy of *Another 9½ Weeks* you've already rented six times this year and tiptoe past the popcorn machine. Don't be afraid. Nothing back there will bite you. Unless, of course, you take that life-size movie poster *Venus Flytrap* seriously. There you go, pull your last leg all the way inside and admire the "colorful" video boxes.

That's okay, everybody smirks at the ridiculous titles. For who could take *Drive Me, Miss Daisy*, *Sinderella*, and *Titanic (Proportions)* seriously. Except their

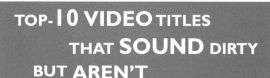

TOP-10 VIDEO TITLES THAT SOUND DIRTY BUT AREN'T

10 **Free Willy**

9 **Deep Impact**

8 **Octopussy**

7 **Lady & the Tramp**

6 **Double Team**

5 **In Too Deep**

4 **The Fly**

3 **Contact**

2 **The Longest Yard**

1 **The Wood**

Need some help? Here's a tip: If you're a guy picking one up for your lady, save yourself a slap in the face and go with erotic or sensual. She'll think you're being "romantic" and trying to add a little "spice" to your romance, and you'll still get to enjoy porn on a weeknight. If you're a lady, however, your man will enjoy the fact that you thought of him and went with raunchy. After all, porn is porn, no matter what the setting. Besides, you wouldn't be back here if you didn't

> "Who needs **him?**
> **I've** got a **vibrator!**"
>
> —Mary Jensen Matthews
> (Cameron Diaz) in,
> *There's Something
> About Mary*

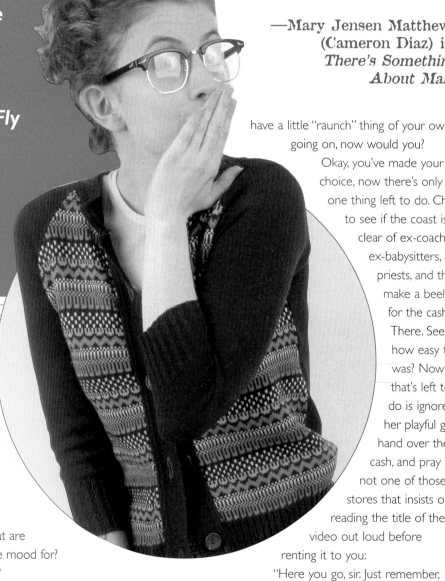

have a little "raunch" thing of your own going on, now would you?

Okay, you've made your choice, now there's only one thing left to do. Check to see if the coast is clear of ex-coaches, ex-babysitters, and priests, and then make a beeline for the cashier. There. See how easy that was? Now all that's left to do is ignore her playful grin, hand over the cash, and pray it's not one of those stores that insists on reading the title of the video out loud before renting it to you: "Here you go, sir. Just remember,

filmmakers, that is. (And even *that's* a stretch.) Sure, you can touch them. With your hands, anyway.

Now, take your time. No need to rush. After all, your old English teacher's still out there among the "mainstream" videos anyway. Now, what are you and your lover in the mood for? Raunchy? Erotic? Sensual?

Sleep Less and Straddle is due back tomorrow before 10 p.m. Enjoy."

Of course, that's fine for so-called "straight couples," but what about same sex couples. Are they to be denied the pleasure of a blissful Blockbuster night simply because they're both named Buster?

Although the "lesbian lovers" section at most video stores is still not quite as large as the new release section (or even, say, karate flicks), couples living an alternative lifestyle, with only a little innovative imagination, can enjoy a plethora of gender-bending (or at least gender-stretching) movie rentals until the rest of the world catches up with them and gives them the floor space they deserve.

The movie *Ghost* immediately springs to mind. Not only is it likely to be in the video store's 49 cent "old release" section (or, if you prefer to own, the $6.99 clearance aisle down at Wal-Mart), but both of its stars cross genders naturally and, one assumes, quite unintentionally.

Jack Daniel's-throated since her early days as an ace journalist on *General Hospital*, the ever-tough Demi Moore sports a *Karate Kid* "bob" and it's pretty clear that ever since *Dirty Dancing*, most of us just assume Patrick Swayze prefers pink to blue ballet slippers (despite his sexy wife).

Top Gun is another '80s blockbuster that seems destined to become a classic for both male and female "longtime companions." After all, doesn't Kelly McGillis' name pop up in most lesbian conversations? And the day Tom Cruise and Val Kilmer both come out of the collective closet will either be a cause for great celebration (or mourning) around the globe.

"**Hell** hath no **fury** like a **woman** scorned for **Sega**."

—Brodie (Jason Lee) in, *Mallrats*

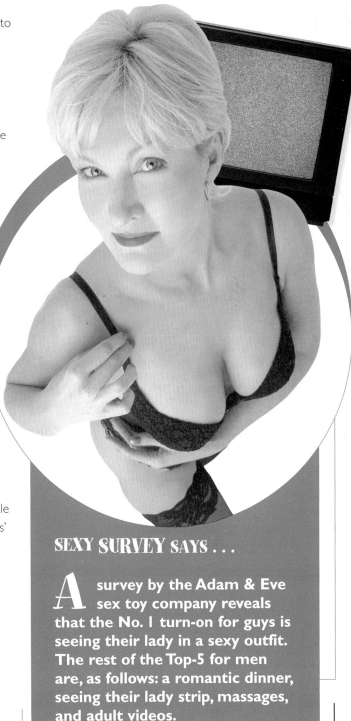

SEXY SURVEY SAYS . . .

A survey by the **Adam & Eve** sex toy company reveals that the No. I turn-on for guys is seeing their lady in a sexy outfit. The rest of the Top-5 for men are, as follows: a romantic dinner, seeing their lady strip, massages, and adult videos.

BIG VS. LITTLE
(SCREENS, THAT IS...)

So, let's see, you're making the big bucks now. Right? Or, at the very least, you have just enough credit left to finally push you over the "Chapter 11 is for losers" threshold. You've got the leather couch, the funky, odd-angled, bi-level coffee table, the Pottery Barn candles that smell like peach and almonds, and if that Ficus plant in the corner was any healthier it would scream, "Feed Me!" three times a day. There are enough throw pillows in your living room to fill a corn silo, your coasters are imported marble, and your Euromassage recliner does things to your backside that are illegal in at least ten states.

So why settle for a 19" TV screen? After all, weren't you thinking about investing in one of those rooftop satellite dishes so you can get that new digital cable package you read about in the paper last week? You know, the one with 180 channels, 60 of which are premium, 24 of which are "adults only," 12 of which are sports, 9 of which are food, and one of which is nothing but 24-hour weather reports from Venezuela.

Now, do you want to watch all of that prime-time entertainment on a screen the size of your computer monitor? Didn't think so. Okay, let's consider your numerous hi-tech home-theater options. There's satellite. There's pay-per-view. There's cable. There's digital cable. There's digital cable via satellite with the optional pay-per-view package.

There's projection screen, wide screen, giant screen, jumbo screen, and even flat screen. You've got your surround sound, picture in picture, sleep timer, and an all-in-one remote control that does everything but put the Orville Redenbacher Light popcorn in the microwave for you. And all for just under the price of one of those new Mercedes SUVs.

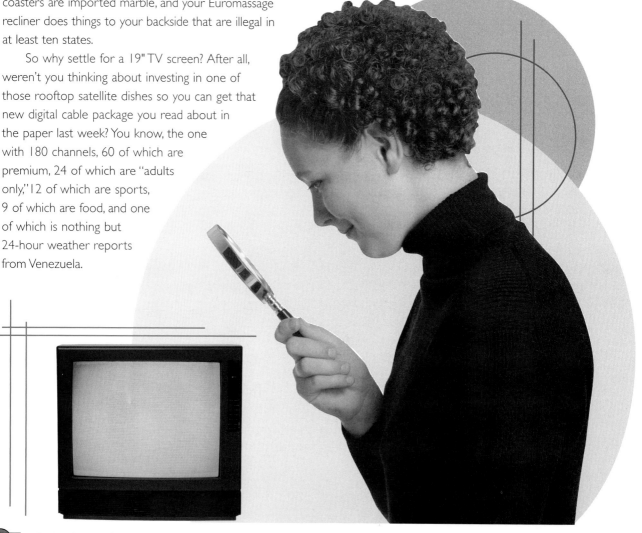

TOP-5 WAYS TV IS BETTER THAN THE MOVIES

5 No line in the restroom. (Unless your boyfriend had Mexican food!)

4 Try fast-forwarding through *Runaway Bride* at the theater!

3 At least that sticky stuff on the floor is your spilled soda.

2 It's much easier to sneak junk food in.

1 The only jerk throwing popcorn at your head is your girlfriend.

Now, before you commit to such an expensive purchase, you want to make sure it's worth the money. Right? Naturally, we're not talking about cathode ray tubes and head cleaners here. We're talking about optimum performance, as in, "Will all of this hi-tech, hi-resolution, hi-end equipment pay off where it really matters . . . with the opposite sex?"

The answer, of course, depends on how you utilize your . . . equipment. After all, no matter how many chick-flicks you agree to see at the theater, your girlfriend, date, or significant other will eventually pine for a soap opera

setting that's a little more intimate. And no matter how many gory, blood-soaked drive-ins you endure, even the most die-hard boyfriend will yearn for the days when he doesn't have to walk the length of a football field to use the restroom.

Therefore, the well-equipped "home theater" can be that all-important "next step" in a healthy, modern couch potato relationship. Why, with so many channels, it's simply a matter of "question and answer" before hitting on a winning combination that any modern single might find hard to resist. Is he a golf nut? Then simply point to the 32 conveniently highlighted (by you) sports channels in your phone-book-sized *TV Guide*. Is she a hopeless romantic? Just casually mention the Danielle Steel marathon currently swooning across any and all of your 12 "Women's Channels." Conveniently forgetting to mention, of course, the 10 "Men's Channels," you wouldn't want her to know about just yet.

Of course, there has always been a huge difference between

the bona fide, sitting-in-a-movie-theater summer blockbuster and a Blockbuster night. While the former involves large crowds and little occasion for actual intimacy, the latter is quite the opposite.

For one thing, there is the slightest hint of a "power play" going on here. Many couples even go so far as to meet at a movie theater for their very first date. This clever tactic, of course, provides a certain amount of freedom and, more important, an escape valve should he turn into a nose-picking slob or she should turn into a "talker."

The home theater, of course, provides none of these escape valves. Hence, whoever is hosting the evening, whether male or female, holds most of the power. They have usually chosen the videos, cooked or at least ordered-in the dinner of their choice, and you have had to drive to their house, apartment, suite, loft, flat, bunker, or basement.

From the minute they open the door and welcome you inside, therefore, the focus is on you and your unspoken laziness. "After all," your host implies but doesn't actually say, "I've done all this work, all you've done is show up!" Internally, this provides the guest with a guilty feeling that often lends itself to thoughts of repaying one's host. Traditionally this token of one's esteem has been a sexual favor of some sort, whether it be a goodnight kiss or breakfast in bed the next morning.

Of course, coming to the door with a good bottle of wine can instantly assuage such feelings. But then, common sense and romance are roads that rarely meet. Instead, an evening is spent in front of the flickering television screen, though neither half of the couple actually watches, listens to,

TOP 5

TV CHANNELS SURE TO DRIVE HIM STRAIGHT INTO THE BEDROOM (TRUST US!)

5. The Food Network
4. Bravo
3. Lifetime, Television for Women
2. Romance Classics
1. A & E

TV CHANNELS SURE TO DRIVE HER STRAIGHT INTO THE BEDROOM (TRUST US!)

5. The Weather Channel
4. ESPN
3. Nickelodeon
2. Playboy TV
1. The Golf Channel

or even cares what is going on in front of them.

All of the action, so to speak, is on the couch, sofa, love seat, or futon.

Distance between the cautious couple is the premium of this relationship, of course. As the host is more often than not the pursuer in this game of cat and mouse, the onus is on him or her to bridge this distance. In the most socially appropriate manner, of course.

Most often this distance is closed by various hostly gestures that are really well, or-not-so-well, camouflaged ploys. Forgetting the microwave popcorn in the kitchen is a classic move, earning the host several inches on his return as he places the popcorn in a better position for her grasp.

She may forget the wine or wine glasses, thus returning to the kitchen and back again, picking up as many comfortable inches as she dares upon her return. Bathroom trips, ringing phones or doorbells, lowering or raising the air conditioning, swatting flies, or even feeding the cat are all opportunities to rise from one's seat half a couch away and return half a foot closer.

Despite how much distance one is able to gain, however, body language, as always, is the key to deciphering your date's desire level. A date who shows more interest in his popcorn (which just happens to be located next to your knee) is obviously ready to "fast forward." If a girl keeps turning the sound down each time you clear your throat, she is more interested in the lame lines you're spewing than the dialogue on the screen. Naturally, these are the "good" signs.

"Bad" signs include a date who's glued to the screen and who, each time you open your mouth, says things like, "I wonder what the characters are saying," or "Look, I came here to watch the movie. You know how hard it is to get a copy of this right now? It's a new release!"

Of course, Blockbuster nights are always a gamble. And, just like other forms of gambling, there are good

and bad outcomes. Then again, there are the longshots.

These include the guy who shows up with flowers, wine, chocolate, and a pleasant patter so smooth and easy you can't remember what happened between the previews and the closing credits. Or the girl who shows up with the kind of

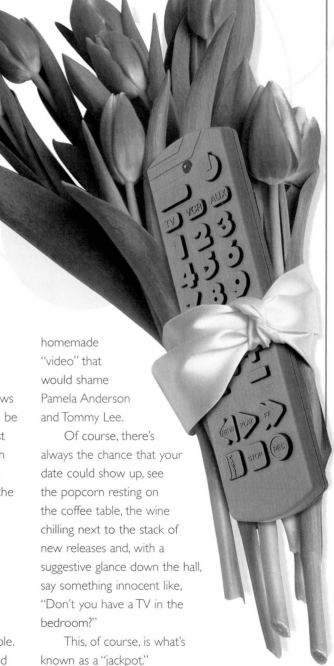

homemade "video" that would shame Pamela Anderson and Tommy Lee.

Of course, there's always the chance that your date could show up, see the popcorn resting on the coffee table, the wine chilling next to the stack of new releases and, with a suggestive glance down the hall, say something innocent like, "Don't you have a TV in the bedroom?"

This, of course, is what's known as a "jackpot."

TICKET TO DISASTER: YOUR FIRST FOREIGN FILM

"I like two kinds of men: domestic and foreign."

—Mae West

SHE SAID

Lana needed answers. Serious answers that she didn't have the courage just yet to ask out loud. "Does he love me? Like me? Is he still interested in me? Is this relationship based on more than just sex? Will he come if I call?"

So she did what every hot-blooded American woman through the ages has done. She combed the highbrow Arts & Entertainment section of the local Sunday paper until she found the most hideous sounding foreign film she could find, and then bought two tickets.

The following weekend, Lana and her unsuspecting boyfriend, Kyle, enjoyed their usual Saturday night date dinner at a local bistro downtown, pleasantly earthy and filled with local eccentrics, but not quite dangerous. When he began lingering over his second cup of coffee, she quickly signaled the college waitress and paid the bill.

Kyle took notice at that, however, and was instantly suspicious. "Hey, what's going on here?" he asked, annoyingly tinkling his spoon against the side of his coffee cup for the thousandth time, or so it seemed to Lana. "Did I forget our first-date anniversary again?"

Lana held firm and whipped out the snooty looking movie tickets from her tiny, sequined purse. "Nope," she said innocently. "I just want to get to the movie theater on time."

Kyle relaxed. He'd seen the "Arts" section of the Sunday paper still lingering on the coffee table all week, and had been afraid that she'd want to go to the opera or some other boring torture chamber. But dinner and a movie he could handle.

Lana even offered to drive, another clue that something was not quite right. Still, Kyle relaxed in the passenger seat, contentedly munching on stale mints from the restaurant and only becoming alarmed when she swiftly passed the multiplex parking lot up the road and soon turned down a deserted street known mainly for its art galleries and wine tastings.

"Lana," he said as casually as possible. "You just passed the movie theater back there."

"That's not the only movie theater in town, Kyle," she sighed, trying to remember the address from the front of the two movie tickets.

HE SAID

Kyle perked up in his seat, wondering if Lana had been reading *Cosmopolitan* again and found a little out-of-the-way adult movie theater on the off chance that it might add a little thrill to their decidedly average sex life.

Alas, while the theater was certainly out of the way, it was also *trés* adult, as in, boring. There wasn't a neon sign to be had, and he couldn't make out any of the words on the tattered movie posters.

"Lana?" he asked hesitantly as she pulled into a mostly empty parking lot. "Is this a surprise party or something? A gag?"

"Not at all, Kyle," she said defensively. "I thought I'd

add a little culture to our weekend."

After that, of course, Kyle whined all the way to the ticket booth. Not only was he not seeing a XXX movie, like he had so briefly hoped, but he wasn't even seeing a movie in which they spoke English! Lana handed over their two tickets to *Nostradamus Portabello* and there was absolutely nothing he could do about it.

When she saw the expression on his face, she went at him loaded for bear, "I can't remember how many stupid sports bars I've been dragged to on a Sunday afternoon or Monday night to watch your stupid football games. The least you can do is spend a measly three and a half hours reading subtitles with me in this quaint little movie theater. I hear *Nostradamus Portabello* is one of the finest films to come out of Pakistan this year."

Her voice thundered through the empty lobby, yet the anorexic artist type behind the concession stand merely glanced up from his tattered copy of Ayn Rand's *Fountainhead*. Obviously he'd heard this speech before.

"Okay, okay," Kyle soothed her, taking out his wallet and buying her an almond covered muffin and cup of espresso (they didn't even serve junk food, for goodness sake) as a peace offering. She smiled, and they proceeded into the darkened theater. Once settled, Kyle was surprised with the comfort of the ancient theater's battered orange chairs and with how much room he had to spread out his long legs. He even liked the antique sconces on the walls and admired the intricate molding on the ceiling tiles while Lana complained about the place smelling like a monkey house at the zoo and wondering why her shoes kept sticking to the floor.

Kyle suppressed a tempting "I told you so," and dove into his cranberry butter scone and frozen mocha frost. The previews silenced Lana's grumblings and Kyle took the reading glasses he rarely used (on a date night anyway) out of his shirt pocket as *Nostradamus Portabello* began grandly on the movie screen.

He was surprised by the fact that the film was actually in color and that it had sound. Of course, the people spoke a different language, but big white letters in a little black box at

TOP-5 EXCUSES TO GIVE FOR NOT GOING TO A FOREIGN FILM

5 Your parole officer frowns on your imagination leaving the country.

4 It's your turn to delouse the cat.

3 Your suicidal religious cult leader forbids it.

2 You're not allowed to miss anymore Charles Manson Fan Club meetings.

1 Your house arrest collar only allows you to go to domestic films.

the bottom of the screen told him what they were saying. Still, he found it a challenge at first to keep up with them, especially with Lana whining right next to him the whole time.

"What did that say?" she kept asking. "These subtitles move way too fast. Did you see a manager out front? Someone needs to complain."

Kyle knew, of course, that that "someone" meant him, but he was too engrossed with the moving story of Nostradamus and his doomed mushroom field to even think about leaving now. Eventually Lana calmed down, but she never quite bought into the story of the dowdy psychic and his depressing portabello predictions.

She leaned her head on his shoulder and, shortly thereafter, didn't even wake up when Kyle snatched her uneaten muffin.

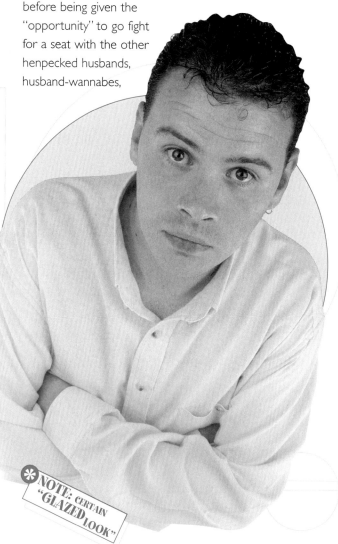

THE **FIVE** LEAST PAINFUL FOREIGN FILMS **YOU** CAN RENT

5 *Cinema Paradiso*

4 *Farewell My Concubine*

3 *Il Postino*

2 *Life Is Beautiful*

1 *Belle de Jour*

"You don't tell a woman that you love her and then two days later bring Romeo over to sleep with him!"

—Nina (Jennifer Aniston) in,
The Object of My Affection

DISPATCHES FROM A CHICK-FLICK/ACTION FILM HOSTAGE, OR: SCORING POINTS THE EASY WAY

HE SAID

It's a certain *glazed look, recognizable from blocks away. A look that can only be called, "trapped." Trapped, that is, in the chick-flick line.

For it's one thing to casually mention, usually just before sex: "Yes, dear, of course I'll go see that new Julia Roberts/Richard Gere romantic comedy with you." Yet it's quite another to actually have to stand in line before being given the "opportunity" to go fight for a seat with the other henpecked husbands, husband-wannabes,

* NOTE: CERTAIN "GLAZED" LOOK

or husbands-in-training to view the film.

Of course, while standing in line waiting to go see the dreaded chick-flick, one gets to see all the other guys inhaling bags of popcorn and Twizzlers on their gleefully unattached way into the latest shoot 'em up thriller, which just happened to open to rave reviews (in *Slaughter* magazine, anyway) on the very same weekend.

A guy can only compare it to the feeling he had when he was sick in bed as a youngster and had to spend the entire day tossing a baseball up and down in a useless mitt while the rest of the team ran off to a big game down at the ballfield.

In such matters, once a suitable grieving period is observed, of course, an ambitious male suitor can turn this huge negative into an even larger positive. For, after all, appearances are everything. You, as the male, are given credit just for showing up, keeping your promise, and not acting like a big crybaby and faking a headache or other invisible ailment just to get out of it. That being said, of course, anything else is fair game once you are actually at the theater.

Or even before you get there, for that matter.

> "I'm goin' to Greece for the sex. Sex for breakfast, sex for dinner, sex for tea, and sex for supper."
>
> —Shirley Valentine (Pauline Collins) in, *Shirley Valentine*

First of all, since the movie will undoubtedly suck anyway, you can allow her to take all the time in the world getting ready. (Thus earning points just for being "patient.") Also, you can graciously offer to escort her to her seat since she made you late (more points for making her feel guilty) and now it's dark and the previews have already started (which earns you major points for being a gentleman).

And, since you certainly don't mind missing the beginning (not to mention the middle or the end) of the movie, you can ask her what she'd like from the concession stand (earning you points for thoughtfulness). Furthermore, you can ask her to tell you what happened while you were gone—earning you double bonus points for, a.) being easygoing and, b.) listening to her when you get back! Your points at this stage are quickly approaching astronomical proportions!

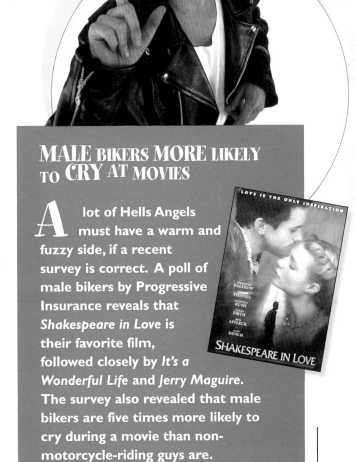

MALE BIKERS MORE LIKELY TO CRY AT MOVIES

A lot of Hells Angels must have a warm and fuzzy side, if a recent survey is correct. A poll of male bikers by Progressive Insurance reveals that *Shakespeare in Love* is their favorite film, followed closely by *It's a Wonderful Life* and *Jerry Maguire*. The survey also revealed that male bikers are five times more likely to cry during a movie than non-motorcycle-riding guys are.

SHAKESPEARE IN LOVE

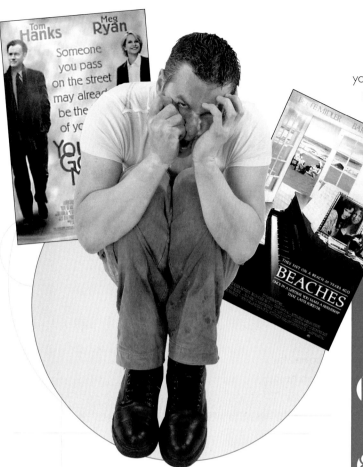

you points that accumulate nearly exponentially the longer you are away.

Upon returning after nearly thirty minutes in the "bathroom," of course, her maternal instincts are hopefully in high gear and, if you are lucky and she is sane, she quite possibly will offer to drive you home right

TOP-10 CHICK-FLICKS TO IMPRESS YOUR GIRLFRIEND (*TRUST US*):

10 *While You Were Sleeping*

9 *You've Got Mail*

8 *Moonstruck*

7 *Sleepless in Seattle*

6 *Pretty Woman*

5 *When Harry Met Sally ...*

4 *Steel Magnolias*

3 *Waiting to Exhale*

2 *The Way We Were*

1 *Beaches*

Of course, she'll never know that you popped into the latest car chase, shoot 'em up, T & A filled thriller in the theater right next door. Even if it is just to stand there inside the lobby and soak up as much gratuitous sex, burnt rubber, and violence as you can before grudgingly leaving the "good" theater to rush to the concession stand, fill her order, and race back to the "bad" theater to endure even more self-induced chick-flick torture.

Of course, if you order the right items at the concession stand, you can miss even more of the intolerably sappy melodrama or romantic comedy you plunked down most of a $20 bill for. Nachos, of course, lead to gastric distress in most, if not all, human beings and, whether they have the same effect on you or not, can easily get you a fifteen or twenty minute bathroom reprieve, again, whether you need it or not.

Accordingly, while you while away a few more gaseous yet blissful moments in the neighboring theater, you are getting her sympathy vote, which earns

TOP-5 SIGNS YOU'RE AT A CHICK-FLICK

5 Your girlfriend actually gets ready on time.

4 You miss the "funny" parts because half the audience is still explaining the concept of "sensitivity" to the other half.

3 Gwyneth Paltrow and/or Julia Roberts are in every preview.

2 Your girlfriend can't stop crying; you can't stop puking.

1 None of the other guys will look you in the eye.

SHE SAID:

Hmm, let's see. Infinite bullets flying out of machine guns that miraculously never jam. Car chases for no reason where, magically, no one but the bad guys ever get hurt. Not a single cop around for miles. Endless dark alleys filled with sinister characters. Numerous "I'm taking you off the case" soliloquies. And a fading action star wearing body armor and too much makeup. Yep, you're at an action flick.

Well, it was inevitable. He's been such a good boy lately. Helping you with the dishes. Taking out the trash. Brushing his teeth before bed. (This is your boyfriend we're talking about, right?) So you figure the least thing you can do is sit through one of his moronic movies for a change. After all, he's been begging you to see *Die Hard 14* for months.

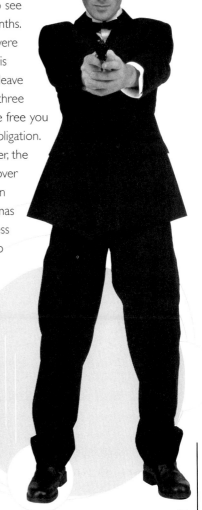

Naturally, you were simply waiting for this miserable bomb to leave the theaters within three weeks and therefore free you from your odious obligation. Miraculously, however, the movie has grossed over eight hundred million dollars since Christmas (it's May, for goodness sakes) and shows no sign of letting up anytime soon.

"But all the other guys have seen it,"

away, seeing as you are so "sick."

No matter how tempting this offer is, of course, you must refuse in order not to lose the impressive score you've built up all evening, which would, after all, instantly reset back to zero by the "wuss" factor (which would make all bets, and future lovemaking, off).

No, you must be "strong," and utter, no matter how nauseating it may be, a line similar to: "No way. I promised you I'd see this movie and I stick to my promises. Besides, now that I'm here, I like it. Really."

Then, of course, as the points pile up like something off of a lotto multiple, she can lean her head contentedly on your chest where, fortunately, she can't see your eyes close as you settle in for a little pre-coital cat nap.

Just don't screw it up and snore.

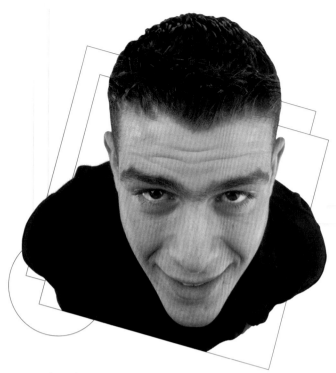

Speeding through yellow lights and cursing little old ladies trying to cross the street, he screeches into the movie theater parking lot in record time. Practically dragging you by the hand, he plunks down an exorbitant amount (shouldn't they give these things away for free? They're so awful!) for your tickets and then buys so much popcorn, soda, and candy you require two trays and the assistance of a burly usher.

"What are we doing here so early?" you ask him once seated and surrounded by greasy popcorn and chocolate covered raisins. "We're the only ones in the theater."

"I was afraid it would sell out," he says pitifully, straining his neck to get a good look at the screen as you grumble about sitting in the third row.

"And explain why we're sitting so close again?" you ask, sipping a soda and wondering if pretending to choke on a licorice whip would somehow get you out of this evening.

he whimpers on Wednesday night with nothing else to do and the movie pages spread out in front of him. "I can't even join in when they're all talking about it. I feel so left out and empty."

Of course, he follows this pitiful statement with an even more pitiful look, the one with the quivering chin and glistening eyes that always makes you want to snatch him up in your arms and hold him tight. Anything, to keep from going to some god awful action flick.

Finally, however, he wears you down. You're fresh out of excuses, he knows it's not "that time of the month" anymore, and your poor grandmother has died more times than that masked guy in *Friday the 13th*! (Please say we're not going to see one of those!)

"Okay," you say, grinning despite yourself to see his face light up like a Christmas tree. "We'll go see *Die Hard 11*."

"Duh," he corrects you, spoiling the mood. "It's *Die Hard 14*. As if."

Naturally, he gets ready in record time and sits waiting by the door like some dog begging to go for a walk. This from a guy who takes half-hour showers and can never remember how to tie his shoes or buckle his belt when you're late for the latest ballet production that's come to town.

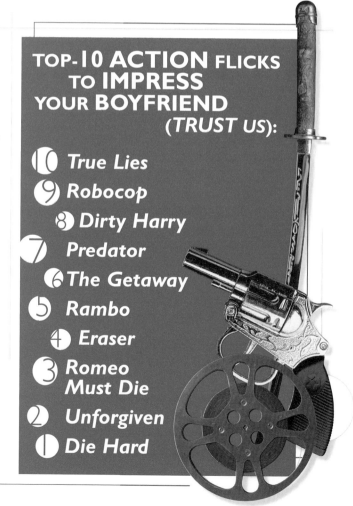

TOP-10 ACTION FLICKS TO IMPRESS YOUR BOYFRIEND (TRUST US):

10. **True Lies**
9. **Robocop**
8. **Dirty Harry**
7. **Predator**
6. **The Getaway**
5. **Rambo**
4. **Eraser**
3. **Romeo Must Die**
2. **Unforgiven**
1. **Die Hard**

"All the special effects," he explains as if to a small child. "You can't really get the full impact unless you sit this close."

Twenty minutes later, the theater is still empty as the house lights go down and your boyfriend of two years (who has suddenly become a complete stranger) taps his foot on the seat in front of you and oohs and aahs at an opening action sequence that finds Bruce Willis climbing a skyscraper with only his bare hands and some silly putty.

"Oh, please," you snort, proceeding to explain the law of physics to your wincing boyfriend. "Everyone knows that bubble gum works much better in that situation."

After shushing you through a mouthful of popcorn and Whoppers malted milk balls, your boyfriend settles into a gunfight that literally lasts ten minutes.

"He's got a pistol and no pockets," you point out gleefully. "Where is he getting all his ammo?"

The movie continues endlessly, but no more so than your insightful comments:

"Do you know how much it hurts to jump through a plate glass window? I do. I saw a special on *Oprah*. He's jumped through sixty-three without a scratch. I've been counting."

"In the last scene, his stolen cop car had a flat. Now he's in Nevada. Do cop cars have double gas tanks?"

"Wasn't he bald in *Die Hard 8*?"

"How funny, his love interest just happens to look like Demi Moore."

And then, an amazing thing happens. Your wish comes true. Out of nowhere, your

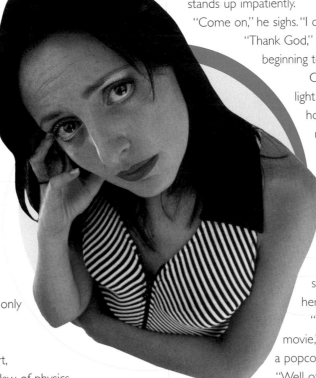

boyfriend bundles up his landslide of snacks and stands up impatiently.

"Come on," he sighs. "I can't take it anymore."

"Thank God," she said. "I was beginning to think I'm dating a moron."

Once in the bright light of the theater lobby, however, you see you've misunderstood him.

"The movie was fine," he explains. "It was you I couldn't take anymore."

"But look," you assert. "I showered. I conditioned. I even shaved my legs. I'm here. What's wrong?"

"You're making fun of the movie," he whines, trying to get at a popcorn kernel with his tongue.

"Well of course I am," you insist. "Why wouldn't I? It's ludicrous."

"Yeah," he says. "But I liked it, and you ruined it for me. Let's just go home."

He looks so disappointed that you feel your heart break, and not just from the sudden popcorn indigestion. Feeling ashamed at your bad movie behavior, you search desperately for a way to make it up to him.

Spotting another movie starting just then at a theater nearby, you suggest giving it a try.

"Only if you promise not to humiliate me anymore," he nearly whispers, defeated.

"I'm sorry," you coo. "I promise."

Perking up, he snatches you inside yet another darkened but empty theater, just in time for yet another opening scene full of gratuitous blood, guts, and gore.

"Wait a second," you finally interject. "What's this one about?"

"Who knows," he smiles. "But Van Damme's in it, it must be good."

Surely, *Die Hard 15* is playing somewhere!

6

LET'S TALK ABOUT SEX!
(OR BETTER STILL, LETS DO IT!)

*V*ery few of us, when asked the eternal question, "How is your sex life?" respond with anything more than, "It could be better." The fact of the matter is, that is usually quite true. You think it could always be better.

Today's hipsters, of course, have a variety of options when it comes to improving their sex life: more partners, better partners, fewer partners, chat room partners, partners of the same sex, partners with cybersex passwords, partners with membership cards to the local "Porn of the Month" club, etc. And whether it's your very first time or your fifteenth one-night stand this month, there's always a new way to spice up your love life. Here's how.

SEX-IQUETTE: YOUR POLITE GUIDE TO ONE-NIGHT STANDS

One-night stands. Don't you just love 'em? The smoky bar. The boozy glance across the smoky bar. The boozy glance across the smoky bar and the extra shot of courage that helps you up off your barstool to ask that Tom Cruise look-alike to dance. Not to mention the asthma attack, bloodshot eyes, and swollen tongue the next morning, accompanied by a massive hangover, bruised toes, and a total stranger lying next to you who looks more like Jerry Springer than Jerry Maguire.

Though the dangers of one-night stands receive the kind of attention reserved for smoking or serial killers, let's face it: They're here to stay. Baptist group scare tactics, sexually transmitted diseases, genital warts, and friends like Linda Tripp have done little to sway America's young, and not-so-young, from getting their jollies the old-fashioned way: one night at a time.

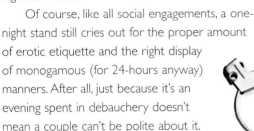

Of course, like all social engagements, a one-night stand still cries out for the proper amount of erotic etiquette and the right display of monogamous (for 24-hours anyway) manners. After all, just because it's an evening spent in debauchery doesn't mean a couple can't be polite about it.

And so, to make such "sticky" social situations just a little less so, we've compiled another helpful guide to ease you through the winding road of one-night stands. Fasten your seatbelts, it's going to be a bumpy ride. (If you're lucky, that is.)

SCORE!

Since we've already supplied you with the goods on everything from kissing to flirting, flowers to secret admirer e-mails, we'll assume that you're already well versed in getting to that all-important stage of picking up the man or woman of your dreams. Chances are, if you're out late enough, still have enough left on your credit card for a nearby hotel room, and have all your teeth, you're going to succeed in scoring a one-night stand *one* of these days.

Accordingly, there are several signs to help clue you in as to this recent development. One of them is the unflinching stare. This is a biggie. Despite your noisy surroundings, "the look" should have a quiet power, and while there's a risk of occasionally lapsing into "spooky," it is generally unmistakable. Naturally, there are two

TOP-5 SIGNS YOU'VE JUST HAD A BAD ONE-NIGHT STAND

5.) Your wallet's empty, your car is gone, and your **kidney's** on its way to **Baghdad.**

4.) You went to bed with **Jerry Hall** and woke up with **Mick Jagger.**

3.) You want to move out; he wants to move in.

2.) The next morning, you get the funniest call from the folks at **Viagra.**

1.) You end up in handcuffs, but not the "fun" kind.

responses to the unflinching stare. One is to look away quickly and change the subject, in which case your ardent admirer will most likely get the picture and turn his or her unflinching stare on the occupant of the very next barstool. The other response is to return the unflinching stare with that other telltale one-night stand sign, the arched eyebrow. This means, "Hey, big eyes, want to see something else grow?"

Another sure sign that your amorous advances are being returned is the exchange of close physical contact. This contact ranges from a light grasp of the arm to both hands desperately squeezing your tight buns, depending on the time of evening and amount of alcohol consumed. Either way, this is the unspoken equivalent of, "Yes, I too would like to enjoy a quiet evening engaging in hot, monkey sex using assorted kitchen utensils."

Other signs include the running of hands through hair (as in, yours), the lighting of cigarettes, the buying of drinks, and the all-around, sure thing, guaranteed one-night stand harbinger, "Did I ever tell you that you look just like the guy/girl who used to live across the street from me growing up?"

Any or all of these signs mean just one thing: Score!

LAST CALL

Naturally, unless you and your passion partner just happen to be among the .0089765 percent of the human population who don't need a quart of gin to walk up to a total stranger and essentially request a passionate evening full of casual sex followed by broken promises and boldfaced lies, most one-night stands

spring from that never ending fountain of youth known as alcohol.

After all, when's the last time you and your accountant had a one-night stand after a long afternoon spent crunching numbers, stubbing out cigarettes, and swilling coffee before your IRS audit? Didn't think so. Therefore, your most likely destination in search of a one-night stand is going to be a bar, café, nightclub, lounge, wedding reception, or, in general, anywhere where alcohol is poured liberally and served frequently.

This, of course, is the beautiful thing about one-night stands. We can always blame them on the alcohol and not our lack of judgment, loneliness, or desperate craving of another human being. Accordingly, neither guilt nor conscience plays a role in such affairs. They are fueled by Jim Beam, stoked by Sam Adams, and slathered in Bailey's Irish Cream.

But just because you're a lascivious lush with mayhem on your mind, doesn't mean that barrooms are immune to etiquette. First off, be prepared. Why do you think there are so many condom machines in bar restrooms? Make use of them. And not just if you're a guy. Wake up, ladies.

If it's 1:59 a.m. and you're the only girl left in the bar, do you really think anyone's going to care whether you stumble into the men's room and pour your last seventy-five cents into the condom machine for a "geisha green" or a "ribbed rainbow?" Chances are you could stumble around during last call picking pockets and tying shoelaces together and no one would notice until they fell ass over trying to pay their bar tab.

Second, be safe. Just because you're about to go home with a complete stranger doesn't mean you should open yourself up to being the main character in Ann Rule's next best-selling true crime novel. Phone a friend and let them know what's going on. Better yet, phone several friends and give them either his address or a phone number where you can be reached. Sure, you may come off as being easy, but what do you care at this point? Weren't you just in the men's room stocking up on condoms and Spanish fly?

THE LONGEST YARD

Following last call, there is the extremely important business of getting home. (Note, this is slightly different from getting to home plate. That comes later.) Naturally, one would hope that if you're inebriated enough to go home with a complete stranger and do unspeakable things with that person on a futon, couch, lawn chair, or kitchen table, that you would still be wise enough to call a taxi.

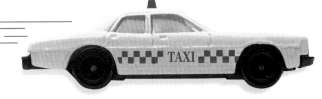

But if you both drove, the question remains, whose car do you take home? His? Hers? Or that new Lexus owned by your "best friend," the one who ditched you hours ago to go home with that hairy dentist at the end of the bar? Either way, certain one-night stand etiquette still applies. For instance, if he drives a hearse, make sure to ride in the front seat. If she drives a Yugo with a missing floorboard on the passenger side, you might want to be a gentleman and offer to drive.

Of course, if your future one-night stand partner is heading straight for that generic white kidnap van you've been seeing all over the news lately, you know,

(Morning, Noon, and) One-Night Stands!

According to a recent public opinion survey on sex conducted by *Bootsy's Sexuality Survey*, how long has it been since you had sex?

	Men	Women
Less than 12 Hours	12%	18%
12 to 24 Hours	13%	14%
1 or 2 Days	18%	15%
3 or 4 Days	14%	9%
5 to 7 Days	11%	9%
8 Days to 2 Weeks	10%	9%
2 Weeks to 1 Month	7%	8%
1 to 3 Months	6%	9%
4 to 6 Months	3%	2%
6 Months to 1 Year	3%	2%
1 to 2 Years	1%	3%
More than 4 Years	2%	2%

the one with the tin-foil covered windows, trailing crime scene tape, and telltale gobs of fingerprint dust, you might just want to call off the whole evening. (Unless you're into that kind of thing.)

Naturally, the smart move in this kind of scintillating situation is to follow each other home. That way, you don't end up in a death mobile surrounded by hanging handcuffs and sharpened door locks. You also have the freedom to bail out at the very last minute should her address be The Seneca School for Schizophrenic Psychos. Also, should you just happen to be listening to Dr. Laura's latest audiocassette tape, *One-Night No No's,* you can always wise up and simply hang left when she's hanging right and just swing by the adult bookstore on the way home. Sure, the live interaction level goes way down, but on the other hand, you arrive alive.

Either way, taking your own car is the best bet. Who knows, you might meet an even cuter guy manning the toll both on the way.

DATING
DESTINATIONS

One-night stands invariably wind up facing one of three occupancy options: his place, her place, or a hotel room. Naturally, all three have their pros and cons. For instance, going back to his place makes great sense for so many reasons. For starters, it means he doesn't ever have to find out where you live. Also, you can feel free to break out the whip cream, chocolate sauce, pickle relish, strawberries, light bulbs, and hamsters without ever having to lift a finger to aid with the cleanup. You can drink his beer, eat his junk food, sweat on his sheets, and, if you get up early enough in the morning, walk away with a brand new stack of souvenir CDs.

On the other hand, if he's the slime ball your mother warned you about, he could be hiding a concealed video camera in the closet. In which case your hidden liaison could wind up in just about every adult bookstore, not to mention cyberporn Web site, across the country. Can you say Pamela Anderson?

Bottom line, it's your call: Free CDs vs. a lifetime of shame and being stopped for autographs by every cybercreep from here to Poughkeepsie.

Going to her house provides another round of copulation chances. For one thing, that annoying smell you haven't been able to get rid of ever since your last crab boil won't present a problem. Likewise, she won't have a chance to run across your shrine to Mötley Crüe. And the fact that you haven't washed your sheets in years won't offend her, either.

Unfortunately, your handy closet full of desirous devices, marital aids, and sexual stimulants won't be at your disposal if you go to her place. Unless, that is, you've thought ahead and stored them in your trunk.

Naturally, there's always that third option of getting a motel room. While relatively expensive, it does spare both of you the option of knowing the other's address, should you consider either one of you to be the least bit schizo. It provides all the cleanliness of her house with the opportunity to be as messy, nasty, and kinky as you want to be at his place, with the promise of a maid coming through the next day to clean everything up, i.e. get rid of the evidence.

Of course, there are other options. If you live in a coastal community, the beach makes a comfy, if sandy, place. If not, how about the local park or ball field? And there's always the backseat of the car.

DIRTY DEEDS
(DONE DIRT CHEAP)

Fortunately, all of your previous etiquette choices fade into the background as the two of you engage in what you've both been anticipating: the actual deed itself. Whether you drove his car back to your place or took a taxi to a room at the local Motel 6, it's not a true one-night stand if either of you are standing. (Unless it's a really *quick* one-night stand, that is!)

Of course, even as the act commences, there's still no reason to be rude. Unless she asks you to do so, of course. Even in the heat of the moment, one-night stand etiquette can still be adhered to.

For starters, try making it to the bed. No matter how difficult this may sound after doing extensive tongue probes at every red light on the way home, not to mention up and down the drive while searching for house keys. Try to make it to the bed. Nothing's worse than the inherent guilt of a one-night stand compounded with the added aggravation of rug burns, waking up with one's hair caught in the shower head, or, worse, one's derriere covered by flour and eggs from a midnight romp on the kitchen table.

Secondly, lose the clothes. Forgetting a cheap earring is one thing, ripping off a silk blouse or mistaking a zipper for a button fly is quite another. However, if you positively, absolutely can *not* wait, at least push up and pull down enough clothing items to leave each and every erogenous zone free and clear of stain-able or dry-cleanable items. Likewise, try to avoid leaving telltale, high school-esque marks on the body, such as hickeys, scratches, or hastily penned marker tattoos containing profanity, phone numbers, or actual names.

> *"Sex is like snow: You never know how many inches you're going to get or how long it will last."*
>
> — Anonymous

(Not Just) One-Night Stand!

According to a recent public opinion survey on sex conducted by *Bootsy's Sexuality Survey*, how many partners have you slept with?

	Men	Women
Zero	7%	8%
1	17%	18%
2	10%	9%
3	8%	8%
4	5%	7%
5	8%	6%
6-10	20%	19%
11-20	10%	15%
21-30	5%	5%
31-40	3%	0%
41-50	1%	1%
51-75	2%	1%
76-100	1%	0%
More than 100	3%	3%

Finally, no matter how repugnant and cheesy you may feel after you've slid into home and dusted off your knees, try and show a little tenderness. Rolling over and going to sleep (aka passing out) may feel like your first initial impulse, but try and fight it if only for a minute or two and give the obligatory hug and, yes, even post-coital kiss. It may not mean you're going steady, but it may just mean the difference between your pocketbook or wallet being twenty bucks lighter the next morning.

(THERE'S GOT TO BE A) MORNING AFTER

Eventually, of course, the passion of the previous evening will pass, the moon will set, the sun will rise, and no matter how hard you try to avoid it, your fluttering eyelids will finally pop open to reveal the lady or lad of the evening snoring peacefully beside you. Of course, if you're lucky and your one-night stand has really been boning up on his or her escapade etiquette, they'll already be gone. Alas, this is mainly the stuff of dreams.

More than likely, the ravishing beauty of the night before will reveal himself or herself to be the ravishing beast that devoured your pillow, not to mention your favorite comforter. Do resist the urge to flee, however. Many an intelligent person has picked up, grabbed what little money they had in their savings account, and simply disappeared off the face of the earth after discovering a previous evening's conquest lolling beside them.

However, entrance into the FBI's witness protection program can be avoided if only a little careful planning is used. This is where being a guy comes in handy. After all, when that comely little lass of the previous night, who has evolved into coyote-ugly a mere eight hours later, asks for breakfast, most guys can simply point to the six-pack of Busch and bottle of ketchup in their fridge and shrug their shoulders.

Girls, don't despair. You too can avoid the dreaded one-night-stand-morning-after breakfast if you'll only wake up early and take advantage of the voluminous space of your dishwasher and oven, most of which are large enough to hold the well-stocked contents of any modern Frigidaire.

And, if the empty refrigerator ploy doesn't work, at least hide your coffeemaker. Even the most malingering morning mates are bound to hit the high road once they hear your coffeemaker's been mysteriously "stolen."

If not, you may want to make that call to the FBI while they're brushing their teeth. Just checking their most-wanted list before planning your day together.

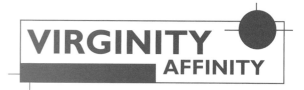

VIRGINITY AFFINITY

Ahh, sex. Whether it's good, bad, or indifferent, sex is an unavoidable fact of life, like death or taxes. (Just a lot more pleasant. Theoretically.) Of course, today, sex comes in a much wider variety than it did for our Biblical cousins. After all, the simple sexual staples of Adam and Eve's day amounted to little more than trying to populate the earth.

Today, however, we have an unending menu of sex, from appetizer to main course to dessert: safe sex, cybersex, kinky sex, fetish sex, interracial sex, transgender sex, same sex, self sex, sex for money, sex for sale, sex for procreation and, our favorite, just plain, good old sex for fun.

Naturally, in this modern world of bare-busted models gracing the covers of grocery store tabloids and kinky keywords typed into computers across the country, sexual awareness starts at a much earlier age than it used to in the good old days of Tom and Huck and Mary Jane. After all, when most of today's techno-savvy shorties are helping the FBI nab prominent public officials by posing as eighteen-year old strippers in the latest strap-on singles chat room, how is playing doctor or spin the bottle supposed to compete?

No longer is sneaking a peak at Dad's collection of dog-eared *Playboys* a thrill. After all, with a ten dollar P. O. Box (half of most kids' weekly allowances these days) and a peek at Dad's credit card number, kids can now have their very own subscription! But why would they need that? After all, with an alarm clock set for 1 a.m. and a remote control, today's techno-savvy junior horndogs can cruise the hundreds of adult channels on their parents' satellite-dish powered TV set and see the real thing in living color. Heck, they can even get it closed-captioned—in Spanish.

Still, while magazines, television, and even cybersex are now staples of most youngsters´, growing up years, the act itself still holds that unique mystique that makes our first time special, no matter how bad, awkward, or messy it may have been. Accordingly, *Buzz On* asks the age-old question:

What Was *YOUR* First Time Like?

ALMOST FIRST TIME

Since I had held out for so very, very, very long (try twenty-five!) to have my first sexual experience, I was hoping that I'd be smart enough to make the most of it. Yeah, right! Although, it started out to be the ultimate first time: The guy was sweet, handsome, charming, gentle, and kind. I'd met him at the library, of all places, doing research on bird watching. He seemed very well informed, but not in an overpowering, know-it-all way. We spent hours buried behind stacks of encyclopedias and bird guides whispering the night away. When the librarian informed us that closing time was quickly dawning, he asked me out for a cup of coffee, and I agreed.

More talking led to an actual date, and several dates later not a single red flag had popped up. The phone number he gave me was actually his. His e-mail address wasn't something stupid like stud69 or idigchicks. He worked at a respectable office, drove a respectable car, and treated me like a lady. So when he asked me over for a nightcap after a lovely, romantic, Saturday night dinner, I assumed I'd be waking up there on Sunday morning.

At first, our nightcap was just that. A little brandy. A little Kenny G on the stereo. (Okay, *one* red flag.) And he kept his distance on the sofa. When he reached out to light a towering apricot aromatherapy candle, however, I couldn't resist any longer and grabbed his paisley tie and pulled him in for one heck of a kiss.

From there it wasn't long until we stumbled, half-clothed, into his bedroom.

And it was there that I found out where he'd been hiding all of his red flags! For starters, there were no less than thirty pictures of his ex-girlfriend who, aside from her dirty blonde hair, looked just like me! Then, there was the huge jar of Vaseline resting on the nightstand where the reading lamp was supposed to be. Not to mention the row of blonde wigs adorning the dresser!

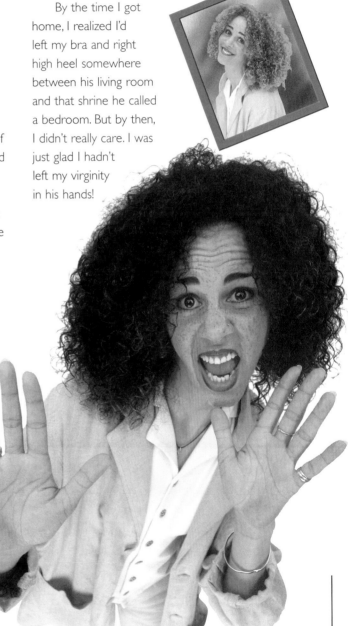

By the time I got home, I realized I'd left my bra and right high heel somewhere between his living room and that shrine he called a bedroom. But by then, I didn't really care. I was just glad I hadn't left my virginity in his hands!

AN OFFER
HE COULDN'T REFUSE

Although I managed to hold on to my virginity all through high school, no easy feat these days, I finally succumbed during my junior year in college. I mean, it wasn't like I was trying to save myself for marriage. After all, who knew if I'd *ever* get married? I'm just really picky. So, when I finally found the right guy, I just went up to him and said, "Hi, my name's Sandra and I've been watching you for months. No, I'm not a stalker. I'm a virgin. Interested?"

Naturally, he was. Not that I'm any beauty queen, but—a virgin's a virgin. And it wasn't like he was a stranger. I meant what I'd said. I really had been watching him for weeks. He was in my Sociology class and I sat in back while he sat up front. I knew every inch of his body (tall, thin, soft), the kind of cologne he wore (Preferred Stock), the style of clothes he liked (Gap vs. Crap), how long he looked at a pretty girl who walked in front of him (just long enough to be hetero, not long enough to be a sicko), and who his friends were (mostly computer geeks, not football jocks who he'd run and blab to the next morning).

YOU KNOW IT'S HER
FIRST TIME WHEN...

5.) She smokes a cigarette **first.**

4.) She comments on how **well**-endowed you are.

3.) She lets you **finish first.**

2.) She asks if you want a beer afterward.

1.) She's afraid to get on top.

I told him exactly how I wanted it to be, and he even picked up half the tab at the drug store, where we bought a cheap bottle of wine, hurricane candles, plenty of bubble bath, and colored condoms. We got a hotel room, turned off the lights, found one of those music channels on the TV, and filled the tub. We started there, but ended up in every inch of the room. It wasn't perfect, but it was perfect for the first time. You know what I mean? I wouldn't have changed it for the world. Except to have bought more condoms, that is.

"Pizza is a lot like sex. When it's good, it's really good. When it's bad, it's still pretty good."

— Anonymous

PSYCHO SEDUCTION

She told me she was a virgin, too. Which is I guess what cinched the deal. I'd been trying to save myself for someone special, but hormones finally got the best of me and by my freshman year in college I couldn't take it anymore. Maybe it was the co-ed dorms. Maybe it was the cheerleaders at all those pep rallies. Maybe it was just the freedom of being away from home. All I know is, by the time I got back from Christmas break, I was about ready to burst.

Fortunately, she had the mailbox next to mine at the student center. I was unloading my fifth load of junk mail into the New Year, and she was unloading hers when we bumped into each other and scattered everything hither and yon. Back then, before my fifth change of major, I was studying to be a psychologist and had just subscribed to *Psychology Today.* When we handed each other back our mail and said good-bye, I thought of her long black hair and even longer legs all the way back to my dorm. And when I lay awake that night tossing and turning, I reached for my new magazine to take my mind off of her "long"-ness and noticed a girl's address on the label on the cover. She must subscribe too!

Racing through the student handbook, I found her name and phone number. I called her the next day to return her magazine. But that wasn't the real reason. It was more of a test. After all, the words in the magazine were the same no matter whose name was on the cover. If she wasn't interested, she could have just said, "Keep it." But she didn't. She acted all surprised and told me to bring it right over.

Of course, romantic that I was, I showered (twice), shaved, and got all dressed up and ran over there reeking of cologne and Dial soap. She answered the door in a silk kimono and before I knew it I was rounding third base and heading for home! Naturally, it was all over rather quickly, and she wasn't exactly the soft and cuddly type. In fact, she did everything but kick me out! Later that day, I realized I never got my magazine back. When I went back to her dorm to retrieve it (and hopefully get lucky again) I noticed some other poor sucker standing at her door with yet another copy of *Psychology Today!*

Hiding behind a potted plant in the lobby, I watched as she opened the door in her kimono, welcomed him in, and then spat him back out exactly fifteen minutes later! I was crushed, and think about her every time I see a copy of *Psychology Today*. Or watch Court TV. Or read a true crime book.

YOU KNOW IT'S **HIS** FIRST TIME WHEN...

5.) He actually holds you afterward.

4.) He says, "I love you."

3.) He says, "I'll never be this good again!"

2.) He lets you finish first.

1.) He says, "No thanks. **Once** is plenty!"

CRABBY LOVER

He seemed like such a sweet guy. But maybe that was just because he was so darned handsome. I mean, this guy's face should be next to the word "dreamy" in *Webster's Dictionary*. I usually don't fall for guys like him, but maybe that was why I finally decided on him to lose my virginity to. Maybe, deep down inside, I knew I'd never meet anybody quite that handsome again. So I let him woo me even though I knew he had a reputation as quite the lady's man. After all, he worked for the same company I did and word gets around fast. Still, it just felt right. He e-mailed me constantly, left funny sticky notes on my computer monitor, and one day he

TOP-5 SIGNS IT'S NOT REALLY HER FIRST TIME

5.) Her collection of autographed *Kama Sutras*.

4.) Keeps saying, "My **last first time** felt better..."

3.) Some guy named **Pimp-Daddy** keeps beeping her.

2.) The clerk at the hotel asks if she wants her **"regular"** room.

1.) Keeps calling you **"John."**

showed up with a picnic lunch (okay, crackers from the vending machine and a Coke) and I just had to say "yes" when he asked me out.

I don't even remember dinner, I was so nervous about what was to come. And, since it was my first time, I wanted it to be in a comfortable place, so I asked him back to my place. Big mistake! Even though the sex was all right, it wasn't quite what I'd expected. Maybe I'd just watched too many skin flicks on *Cinemax After Dark*. He left shortly after it was over and, like a fool, I slept hugging the pillow he'd used and smelling his cologne all night.

Naturally, the next morning I couldn't stop scratching myself. You know, down there? It was like my whole crotch was on fire. I had to leave work before lunch and race straight home, scratching all the way! When I got there, I did a pretty thorough self-examination and finally found what looked like a cross between a tick and a miniature monster from one of those *Alien* movies. Turns out it was crabs! I had to shave, everywhere, delouse everything, and buy all new sheets! I spent

close to a hundred dollars on Rid alone!

Of course, when he finally returned my phone calls, he denied everything and simply told me not to "sleep around" so much. I didn't give him the satisfaction of letting him know he was my first. Instead, I spread a nasty rumor about him at work and watched as it gained ground wildly. Like I said, word spreads fast.

FIRST-TIME FELON

My girlfriend and I had just broken up. She'd been insisting that we save ourselves until we got married, and like a fool, I'd honored her wishes. Then she up and dumped me for the captain of the soccer team and I heard they'd locked themselves in his bedroom and screwed like bunnies for an entire weekend!

Luckily, there was this girl who'd always sort of flirted with me the whole time I was going out with my girlfriend, and like a jerk I called her right after I heard about my ex-girlfriend and the soccer stud. Word was she was sort of "adventurous," and so when she agreed to go out on a date I got a hotel room for later, just in case. Well, the word was right and I don't even think we made it all the way through dinner, she was so revved up. We went back to the hotel room and went crazy with a bottle of wine and the lights off!

When I woke up the next morning, totally hungover, I saw that she was missing. I also saw blood everywhere! I thought I'd gone crazy on a drunken bender and in a fit of jealous rage over my girlfriend stabbed her to death with the remote control! I called her house, I called her friends' houses, I called everywhere and no one could find her.

Finally, just as I was getting ready to flee the country, she came back into the hotel room with a bag full of sanitary napkins and tampons from the drugstore down the street. It seems she'd started her period that night and we were both too drunk to notice!

So, do you still think your first time was that bad?

Didn't think so.

SPICE RACK (OF LOVE)

Well, the good news is you HAVE a love life. The bad news is—it sucks! In a word: lame. In a sentence: the bloom is definitely off. Well, what do you expect? After all, you've already been through that gushing "young love" stage, where you can't keep your hands off each other, let alone each other's private parts. You've made mad, passionate, Discovery Channel love on each and every piece of furniture in your apartment. You've spent entire weekends locked in the bedroom eating nothing but chocolate covered strawberries and drinking champagne. You've written each other wickedly nasty e-mails and actually sent them.

But that was all in the past. Now you're lucky if you have sex at all, let alone on various pieces of furniture or major household appliances. The only e-mails you send anymore are to remind each other to pick up milk on the way home, and the last time you did anything kinky at all was that time the UPS man delivered a box of edible condoms to your door by mistake. Naturally, that was over a month ago.

So what can you do to add a little hard to your hard-drive? A little zip to your zipper? Why not try one (or all, what the heck) of the following tips to add a little spice to your love life. Warning: Intense spice may cause acid reflux of burning passion.

TRICKY STICKIES

If you're looking for a cheap way to inject a little salsa into your bedroom burrito, why not invest in a fifty-nine cent book of sticky notes? At first, it may not appear to be a romantic gesture. But combine this simple purchase with a ballpoint pen (preferably in red) and you've got yourself a powerful aphrodisiac. As long as you can string two words together, that is.

Sure, scribbling "I love you" on a sticky note or two and leaving them on his briefcase each morning is cute.

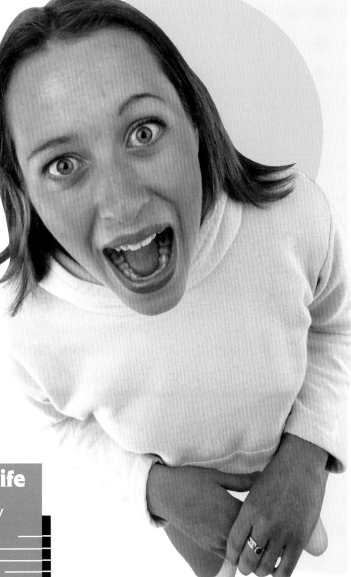

(Spicing Up) Your Sex Life

Have you ever acted out a sexual fantasy with your partner?

No	38%
Yes	62%

[Survey results courtesy of *Women.com*]

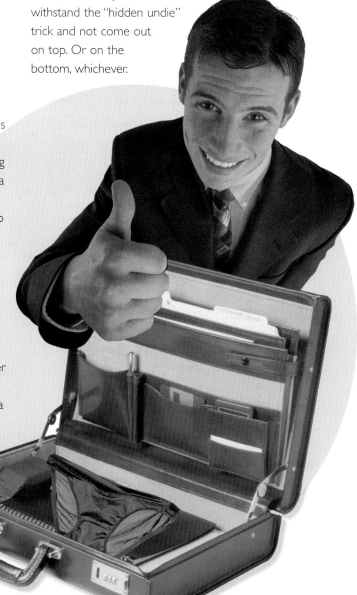

I love your cute little buns!

It may even earn you a surprise kiss on the cheek before you head off to work. But why not go one step further and write him something a little, sexier. As in, "I love your…" Now, you fill in the blanks. (We can't do everything for you!) Your man is sure to love the little added sexiness to his morning coffee, especially if what you love about him lies below his boxers or briefs!

Of course, we can't be responsible for spilled coffee, uneaten breakfasts, broken china, or the two of you being late to work.

Guys, you don't get out of this one either. In fact, you don't even get out of it as easily as the girls did! After all, they expect you to tell them you love their this and thats. (You do that anyway!) No, you get to take those sticky notes and write your lady a love poem that's sure to knock her socks off. Yes, this means you. Don't worry, it doesn't have to rhyme. Doesn't even have to exactly make all that much sense. As long as you write something sweet and spread it out over a week's worth of cuddly yellow sticky notes, say left by her purse or on her pillow each night, you're bound to spice up her week and leave her panting for more.

Poetry, that is. For now, anyway. After all, all good poems must come to an end. And that's where the real fun begins.

UNDERWEAR AFFAIR

Okay, now we're starting to get a little sexier. After all, it's no coincidence that spice and sex both start with the letter "s." Now, this idea requires two things, a briefcase and the purchase of a slinky pair of brand new underwear. Don't worry, the results will be worth it. Chances are, no matter what you buy, you'll never even have to wear them. (Not if this idea works, anyway.)

First, get the underwear. Come on, splurge a little. After all, this is much cheaper than a romantic dinner and loads more fun. Second, buy something that's totally unlike you. If you're a strictly boxer kind of guy, go for the stripper thong. Preferably in electric blue or, for maximum results, zebra skin black and white! Ladies, if you and your grandmother have been buying the same brand of cotton panties for years, why not try a slinky red number that's as see-through as local laws will allow.

Next, get up a little early and slip your pelvis-covering purchase into your lover's briefcase, backpack, or portfolio before he/she rushes off to work. Then sit back and wait for his husky voice on the other end of an unprecedented lunchtime phone call. It's the rare couple who can withstand the "hidden undie" trick and not come out on top. Or on the bottom, whichever.

MASSAGE BARRAGE

Here's another idea that's guaranteed to make skipping the news (not to mention the game shows and sitcoms to follow) an altogether animalistic alternative. First, invest in one of those Sensual Massage guides at the local bookstore. (Not the local adult bookstore. Like we said, that comes later.) Now, bone up on your technique by practicing on a pillow or ironing board before your lover gets home. You don't need a lot of fancy oils, luxurious towels, or New Age music for this one. Simply light a candle or two, make sure the bed is made, and put on your favorite Luther Vandross CD.

Next, welcome your lover home with a sensual massage. A cold beer or glass of wine helps, but is by no means a necessity if you've practiced your technique. Watch as your lover melts beneath your expert hands. Listen as she sighs at your velvet touch. Feel as he squirms beneath you. Then let fate work out the rest. Maybe he falls asleep instantly and wakes you up a few hours later with a massage of his own. Then again, maybe she rolls over and keeps you "up" all night.

Either way, a decent massage is an irreplaceable piece of ammunition in your arsenal of weapons.

WINK, WINK!

This may be the easiest tip to apply, and, surprisingly, the one with the best results. After all, candlelight and soul grooves, massages and erotica are one thing. But a well-timed facial expression can be worth a thousand words. Or grunts and groans, whatever. Kisses are great. Hugs are super. Whispers are nice. Tickles are fun. But let's not underestimate the power of a really good wink.

What's that you say? A wink? Yes, you're reading it right. No typos here. The wink is one of the few remaining mysteries of body language. After all, a wink could mean she's got a hair in her eye and needs medical attention, or it could mean he's dying to give you butterfly kisses all night long.

Of course, a well-timed wink between two lovers

who may have grown a little stale in the bedroom can mean the difference between just another Tuesday night and the kind of midweek passion you'll be telling your grandchildren about when you're a dirty old couple too senile to know any better. Just remember, there's a big difference between a wink and a muscle spasm. One says, "love me." The other says, "help me!"

Trust us, only the first one is sexy. So keep the winking down to a minimum. Still need help? Here are a few times when a nice, well-placed wink can help put you over the edge in his or her heart:

- During a lengthy visit from Aunt Bertha.
- After a news story that says American couples aren't getting enough sex.
- The next time you hear "Afternoon Delight" on the car stereo.
- While you're peeling a banana for his breakfast cereal.
- When you're squeezing melons across from her in the produce aisle.

The rest is up to you. Wink, wink. Nudge, nudge!

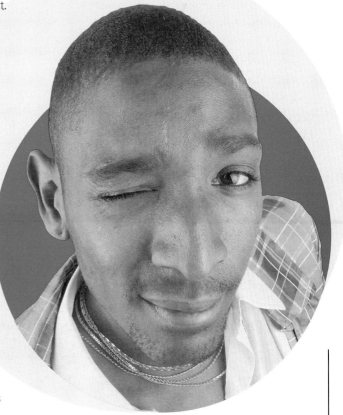

FLOWER POWER

If a wink says a thousand words, then flowers can say a million. That is, if you send or bring them at just the right time. Which does not, we repeat, does not mean after you've had a fight or said or done something incredibly stupid. After all, any dolt can call FTD after staying out too late with the girls from accounting or playing poker well into the dawn with your old college buddies.

The trick is to send flowers for no special reason whatsoever. Sure, it sounds simple. But this timely trick can't work its magic unless you actually remember to do it! After all, you don't need to spend a ton. A bouquet of daisies delivered to her desk at work on some boring old Thursday just to say you're looking forward to another weekend together is sure to make it a weekend worth remembering.

And girls, you're not immune from this one, either. Hey, it's the new millennium. You're allowed to cross the threshold of a florist door yourself now, you know. So do so. Maybe your guy doesn't want a bouquet full of pansies paraded through his office, but a nice potted plant or coffee mug full of miniature cacti is a marvelously macho way to say, "I miss you."

And if you can beat your lover home on the day of your daisy delivery and meet her at the door wearing a pair of gardening gloves and nothing else, your ivy might not be the only thing creeping in her secret garden!

Perky Polaroids

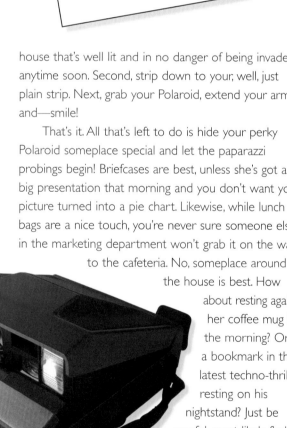

This idea is a bona fide winner, but a tad riskier than all the rest. After all, sending flowers or winking won't get you arrested for indecent exposure. (Unless you do them in the nude in the middle of Main street, that is.) But for this titillating tidbit, you'll need a Polaroid camera and a flexible (preferably double-jointed) arm. First, find a quiet place in the house that's well lit and in no danger of being invaded anytime soon. Second, strip down to your, well, just plain strip. Next, grab your Polaroid, extend your arm and—smile!

That's it. All that's left to do is hide your perky Polaroid someplace special and let the paparazzi probings begin! Briefcases are best, unless she's got a big presentation that morning and you don't want your picture turned into a pie chart. Likewise, while lunch bags are a nice touch, you're never sure someone else in the marketing department won't grab it on the way to the cafeteria. No, someplace around the house is best. How about resting against her coffee mug in the morning? Or as a bookmark in the latest techno-thriller resting on his nightstand? Just be careful, most likely flashes won't be the only things going off in your house. Say cheese!

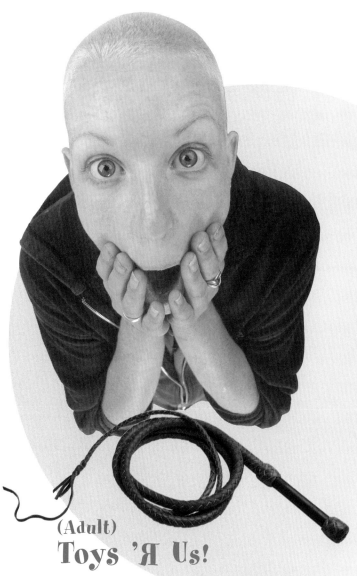

(Adult)
Toys 'Я Us!

Okay, pervs. Here it is. Time for the big blow out. So far we've been spicy, but on a spiciness scale of one to ten, with a wink being a two, this final installment of our spice rack of love is burning up with a sexy score of 2,816, 542!

Now, depending on what city you live in, your local adult toy store could run the gamut from tepid waters to boiling hot! Naturally, for the sake of legality, we're not suggesting full Dominatrix gear or any of that *Pulp Fiction* zippered mask paraphernalia. (We want to spice up your love life, not scare it to death!)

No, we're talking about the fun stuff. Videos and interactive CD-ROMs are fine if you're both into that stuff, but chances are he'll be a little deflated if you bring home *Hung Studs #12* and it's a sure bet that she'll feel less than charitable should you pop in *Big Busted Bombardiers* instead of *The Sound of Music* one quiet Sunday night.

What we're suggesting is just a little on the tamer side. For instance, even though it's not Valentine's Day or a friend's bachelor party, why not stop in on the way home and pick up a pair (or two) of orange-flavored edible panties. Sure, they're cheesy. Sure, they're ridiculous. Sure, they're fattening. But if you stroll in wearing a pair of your own, chances are none of those considerations will even enter the picture. (More pictures. That's a good thing!)

Ladies, where are you going? Adult toy stores aren't just for flashers and dirty old men anymore, you know. Why not surprise your man with a pack of edible condoms? Sure, they may not actually work, but is that really the point? Chances are, one tasty application will make for one fun dessert!

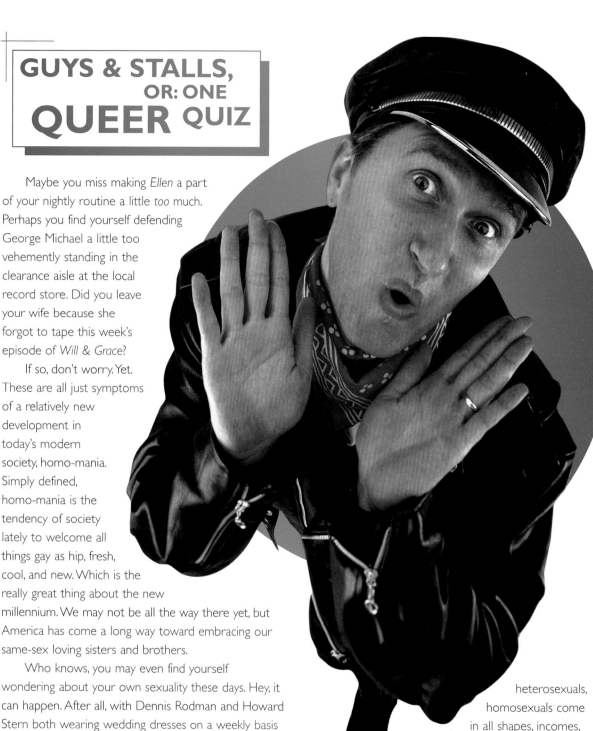

GUYS & STALLS,
OR: ONE
QUEER QUIZ

Maybe you miss making *Ellen* a part of your nightly routine a little *too* much. Perhaps you find yourself defending George Michael a little too vehemently standing in the clearance aisle at the local record store. Did you leave your wife because she forgot to tape this week's episode of *Will & Grace*?

If so, don't worry. Yet. These are all just symptoms of a relatively new development in today's modern society, homo-mania. Simply defined, homo-mania is the tendency of society lately to welcome all things gay as hip, fresh, cool, and new. Which is the really great thing about the new millennium. We may not be all the way there yet, but America has come a long way toward embracing our same-sex loving sisters and brothers.

Who knows, you may even find yourself wondering about your own sexuality these days. Hey, it can happen. After all, with Dennis Rodman and Howard Stern both wearing wedding dresses on a weekly basis and Sharon Stone and Ellen Degeneres making out on HBO, what's the big deal anyway? Is being gay such an odd thing? And if so, why does every news day seem to bring yet another Hollywood hottie or hunk right out of the closet and onto your television screen.

After all, it's not like those ancient stereotypes of yesteryear really apply anymore. We all know that just like heterosexuals, homosexuals come in all shapes, incomes, and bust sizes. The days of butch lesbians and fey queers pretty much bit the dust when we all found out that Rock Hudson preferred Montgomery Clift to Marilyn Monroe. Since then, the parade out of the closet has included the likes of Anne Heche, Rupert Everett, k.d. lang, and Greg Louganis.

So what's to say you're immune? After all, we've all seen those cheesy black and white documentaries on the sexual revolution of the '60s. Bra burning. Divorce. Interracial marriage. Swinger clubs. Legal prostitution. What was once unheard of is now passé. Maybe the recent rash of occupational outings is simply the new sexual revolution and we happy heteros are all just poster children for that most simple of all medical conditions known as denial. (With a capital "D!")

Don't believe it? Well, what's that pile of Indigo Girls CDs doing by your stereo? Or how about that collection of Broadway ticket stubs? At whom do you laugh harder on *Frasier*, Niles or his dad? Does it take you hours just to pick out a simple pair of jockey shorts for yourself because you're so busy ogling the box covers? See what we mean?

Ladies, what is your SEXual Orientation?

Completely heterosexual (no sexual contact with another woman) — **38%**

23% — **Straight, but Bi-curious (willing to try sex with another woman)**

Straight (but have had sexual contact with another woman) — **16%**

Bi-sexual (predominantly interested in men) — **13%**

5% — **Bi-sexual (predominantly interested in women)**

Homosexual — **5%**

[Survey results courtesy of ***Bootsy's Sexuality Survey***.]

If you're still not sure, we have provided you with a little quiz to see whether you're bi, curious, bi-curious, or just plain ready to drop the charade altogether and start wearing chaps. (And we're not talking about the cologne, either!) Ready? Thought so.

1.) First, a question for the guys. Fellas, choose the answer below that best reflects the number of Barbra Streisand albums you own (regardless of the fact that you actually store them at your brother Rob's):

A.) Less than five.
B.) More than ten.
C.) Less then fifteen.
D.) You stopped counting after *The Mirror Has Two Faces* soundtrack.

If you answered "A," rest easy. We all recognize the obvious talent in Barbra Streisand's sumptuous voice and inherent knack for choosing just the right songs for each and every quadruple platinum album. You're nothing more than a happy hetero who's got a lame CD collection. If you answered "B," look out. You are bottom-line borderline. (Especially if one of the CDs is Yentl. *Actually, if one of them is* Yentl, *you can pretty much skip the rest of this quiz and knock on your hunky neighbor's door and ask him out.)*

Of course, if your answer was "C" or "D," you already know something is up. (Unless you were just hired as Barbra's personal assistant and are having a genuine attack of major kiss ass. In which case, we understand.) Naturally, this quiz is considerably less than scientific.

2.) Now for the ladies. Girls, when was the last time you spent the evening perusing through that stack of dog-eared *Playboys* your ex-boyfriend left behind. (And we know it wasn't for the articles!)

A.) Last night.
B.) Last month.
C.) What ex-boyfriend?
D.) What articles?

Now for the results. Ladies, this was a trick question. If you answered any of the above, you are perfectly hetero.

After all, girls have a more open notion about their sexuality. Your sensitivity allows you the confidence to open up a perfectly photographed copy of Playboy, Penthouse, or Swank and enjoy the undeniable beauty of the female form. The tender arc of a graceful thigh. The velvet tones of a freshly shaved armpit. The rosy swell of a budding, swelling, blossoming—hey, stop that! This is supposed to be scientific, not erotic. Maybe you do need to keep reading.

3.) Guys, you're on deck. Pretend your company has just hired a new employee who just happens to be male, extremely, strikingly, model-esque (did we say extremely?) attractive, and assigned to the cubicle next to you. What do you call him?

A.) Whatever it says on his business card.
B.) Dick head.
C.) Pretty-boy.
D.) Big Daddy.

If your answer was, "A," we can pretty much tell you that you're not the warmest person in the world, but you're probably not the gayest either. If you answered "B," we know you're not the warmest person, and can instead tell you that you should lighten up and let the guy enjoy his dashing good looks while they last. After all, beauty fades. (Besides, he's probably not very smart!) Now, if you answered "C," you're either the most straight guy in the world (who doesn't resent a little competition in the workplace? Okay, a lot of competition) or a really big flirt.

Now, unless he's seven feet tall and your father, if you answered "D," we hope you didn't call him that to his face. Unless, that is, the first thing he did at the sight of his new cubicle was gush something like, "I just can't

wait to hang my potted plant there, and won't those twelve pictures of my cat go great there, and, uhhm, this place is just scrumptious." In which case, he probably didn't even answer you at all. (He probably just winked.)

4.) Ladies, we're back to you again. Let's say, just hypothetically, that your old roommate from college calls you out of the blue one day and tells you that she's just come out of the closet. Your first reaction is to:

A.) Tell her she has the wrong number and hang up.
B.) Disguise your voice and ask her what "you" looked like naked.
C.) Cuss her out and blame her for all of your recent problems with men.
D.) Blurt out, "You're so lucky!"

If your answer was "A," congratulations. You just ruined a years-old friendship because you're a raging homophobe. How do you feel now? On the flip side, the good news is you have one less Christmas card to write next year. Of course, if you answered "B," this just goes to prove that you're too vain to love anybody else in the first place, woman or man. Answer "C" is another tough one. For one thing, you sound like a big man-hater. Then again, you sound like a big woman-hater too. So you're probably safe.

Answer "D" is slightly more telling. If you chose this option, you meant one of two things. One, that she's so lucky to finally be free of the oppression of keeping a life-long secret, and she can now live life the way she was meant to live it, happily and out in the open. Two, you're jealous that she's brave enough to admit she prefers breasts to chests, while you are still hopelessly mired in chasing down loveable losers of the male variety. Either way, we hope you got her phone number.

5.) Now for a unisex question. Let's say a member of the same sex asks you out. Just out. Nothing romantic. No flowers and candlelight. Just out to "get to know you a little better." Do you:

A.) Freak out and make some
    lame excuse.
B.) Agree readily, then back out at the
    last minute.
C.) Agree, then stock up on Mace and
    athletic supporters.
D.) Buy new underwear and pack an
    overnight bag.

If your answer was "A," relax. You are a typical, paranoid, delusional, anal American just like your friends and all their friends. After all, what would it look like, the two of you sitting there having dinner? Alone? On a Friday night? Everyone would think you're on a date anyway, right? Even if you weren't. So you had to make up some excuse. Right? On the other hand, maybe your great aunt really did just pass away. (Again.)

If your answer was "B," you could be bi-curious. Then again, you could just be bi-polar. Who knows, maybe you're the same way with friends of the opposite sex. Answering "C," however, indicates that while you're not exactly ready to pitch for the same team, you're at least willing to sit in the dugout and check out his or her swing. Good for you. Now, answering "D" can only mean one thing: You're easy.

So, see there. Our "queer quiz" was relatively painless and hopefully enlightening. Maybe you've cheated and satisfied yourself that you're as straight as Cary Grant. (Whoops.) Then again, maybe you've been honest enough to realize that, while you do have an open mind and don't resent those happy homosexuals their alternative lifestyle, you're just as happy in your own heterosexual skin. Then again, maybe you never even finished the quiz in the first place, you were so busy flirting with that same sex sizzler sitting across from you in the bookstore!

Naturally, this is just an informal quiz to help you see that there's no shame in being homosexual, heterosexual, or a little bit of both. After all, it's a big, big world and love comes in all shapes and sizes, not to mention sexes. Who is to say your soulmate isn't just around the

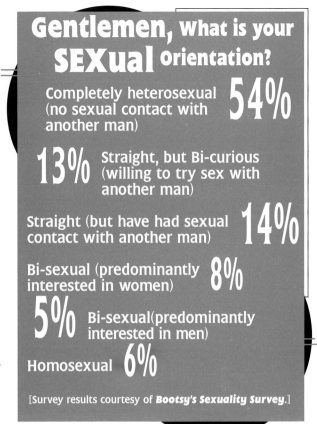

Gentlemen, what is your SEXual Orientation?

Completely heterosexual (no sexual contact with another man) **54%**

13% Straight, but Bi-curious (willing to try sex with another man)

Straight (but have had sexual contact with another man) **14%**

Bi-sexual (predominantly interested in women) **8%**

5% Bi-sexual (predominantly interested in men)

Homosexual **6%**

[Survey results courtesy of ***Bootsy's Sexuality Survey***.]

corner, wearing the same cowboy boots or silk blouse that you are?

After all, this can only mean that you're well on your way to a wonderful life together. For not only do you have the same taste in sexes, but the same taste in clothes as well!

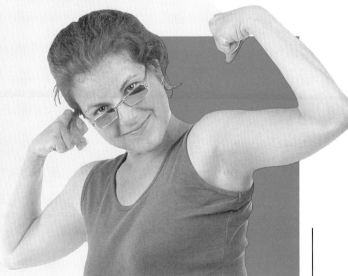

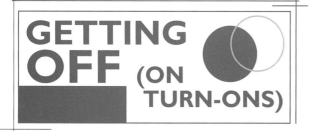

GETTING OFF (ON TURN-ONS)

Ahh, the mating mystery that is sexual attraction. What's hot? What's not? What gets you (off)? What sets you running (away)? Well, as we all know, the answers are as different as night and day. (Or, in sexual parlance, as different as "midnight missionary" or "afternoon delight!") While one finicky female may be fond of guys who are tall, dark, and handsome, her best friend may like them short, darker, and from Sing Sing! Some guys are breast men, some go for thighs. (Yeah, right. We all know most go for both!)

Some ladies love to laugh at the cute class clown, others like the strong, silent type. A lot of guys like a girl who'll listen, some just get turned on by the sound of a sexy voice. (Hey, who do you think is calling all of those 1-900 numbers?)

Red hair. Big hands. Clean teeth. Body hair. Lipstick. Glasses. White hose. Garters. High heels. Tube socks. There are as many variations of turn-ons as there are sexual positions in the *Kama Sutra* and, like snowflakes, no two people respond the same way to the same stimuli. (Unless it's in *Playboy*, that is.)

Some turn-ons are visual. Take small breasts or hairy knuckles, for instance. Some are tactile. Think soft silk or cold leather. Some are auditory. As in, the sound of smooth jazz or numerous zippers unzipping. Some are located on the taste buds. How about whipped cream and strawberries? Naturally, both are twice as stimulating when eaten off of a washboard stomach. However, all turn-ons are unique to the turn-on-ee.

After all, what works for your friend

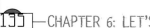

rarely works for you. And if it does, maybe you two should consider becoming more than just friends. Indeed, many people fail to recognize turn-ons when they see, feel, touch, taste, or hear them. ("Wow, I just thought everyone got hot flashes looking at butterscotch pudding!") However, even those who do recognize their turn-ons don't always have the opportunity to act on them. For instance, those who can only get turned-on by skydiving naked on Christmas morning in the rain wearing red leather go-go boots don't exactly have a plethora of opportunities to get turned-on. Likewise, acting on every day turn-ons such as stop lights, cigarette lighters, and Big Macs might get you in a lot of trouble.

But what happens when the very thing your lover thinks will turn you on is the one thing guaranteed to turn you off? "Zip" through the following story and find out for yourself:

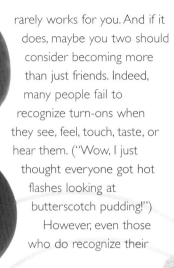

THE QUICKER ZIPPER UPPER

It's been a couple of weeks and all of your dates have progressed naturally and smoothly toward the ultimate goal: sex. (Specifically, hot-buttered, sweaty, funky, monkey lovin'!) You'd played sufficiently hard to get and he'd been sufficiently (if impatiently) patient.

There'd been dinner and a movie, a group date, a sporting event to prove your good intentions, and even a trip to the local playhouse to prove his. But now it was just the two of you at a romantic restaurant. There'd been flowers, candlelight, string music, and good wine.

TOP-5 SLOGANS YOU DON'T WANT TO SEE ON YOUR BOYFRIEND's UNDERWEAR

5.) "Property of State Correctional Facility."

4.) *Batteries **not** included.

3.) "I'd rather be wearing panties."

2.) "Yes, this is as good as it gets."

1.) *Magnifying glass not included.

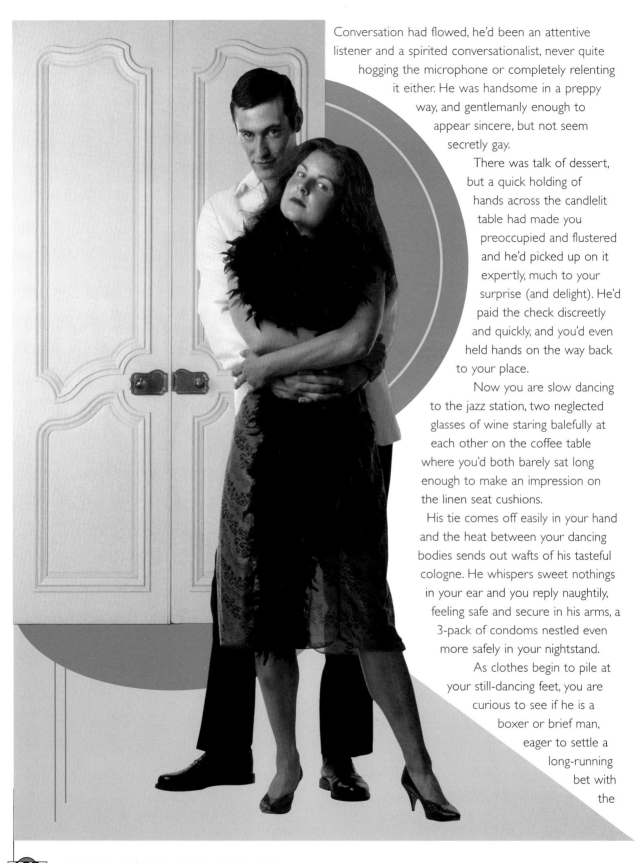

Conversation had flowed, he'd been an attentive listener and a spirited conversationalist, never quite hogging the microphone or completely relenting it either. He was handsome in a preppy way, and gentlemanly enough to appear sincere, but not seem secretly gay.

There was talk of dessert, but a quick holding of hands across the candlelit table had made you preoccupied and flustered and he'd picked up on it expertly, much to your surprise (and delight). He'd paid the check discreetly and quickly, and you'd even held hands on the way back to your place.

Now you are slow dancing to the jazz station, two neglected glasses of wine staring balefully at each other on the coffee table where you'd both barely sat long enough to make an impression on the linen seat cushions.

His tie comes off easily in your hand and the heat between your dancing bodies sends out wafts of his tasteful cologne. He whispers sweet nothings in your ear and you reply naughtily, feeling safe and secure in his arms, a 3-pack of condoms nestled even more safely in your nightstand.

As clothes begin to pile at your still-dancing feet, you are curious to see if he is a boxer or brief man, eager to settle a long-running bet with the

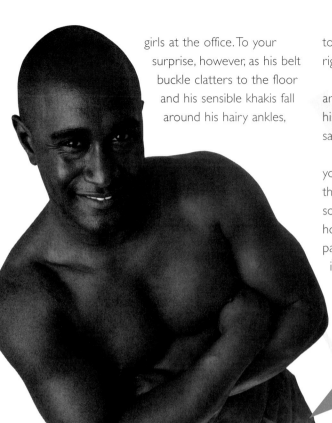

girls at the office. To your surprise, however, as his belt buckle clatters to the floor and his sensible khakis fall around his hairy ankles, you see that he is neither.

He is, in fact, one of those rare (but not rare enough) breeds known as a "jockey jokester." A man so at ease with his sexuality and so confident in his bedroom prowess that he finds the need to search high and low for underwear that is not only colorful but "off-color" as well. Naturally, he considers such cotton come-ons as tantalizing turn-ons. (Never suspecting, of course, the fact that *you* don't!)

Standing back to read the words emblazoned across a barely noticeable bulge, you reach for that forgotten glass of wine and take a healthy drag, if only to have something in your mouth to keep from laughing.

An arrow to the left of his thigh points, of course, to what lays nestled safely inside. A legend to the right reads, "Blow here for a higher I.Q."

Wine be damned, your laughter spills out around the lipstick stained rim, bringing a smile to his suddenly very un-preppy face. "So," he grins satisfactorily, "you like what you see."

"I don't know," you grin. "That depends. That *is* your only pair of those, right? I mean, you bought those as a gag for our big night or, even better, someone gave you them back in high school, your house recently burned down, and they were the only pair you grabbed on your way out the door because it was all cloudy and smoky. Right? Please say 'yes'!"

"No way, baby," he says. "Stick with me and you'll see plenty more funny underwear sayings where this one came from."

"No I won't," you correct, kicking him out the door with barely enough time to cover his jockey shorts joke … not to mention, his unfunny underwear!

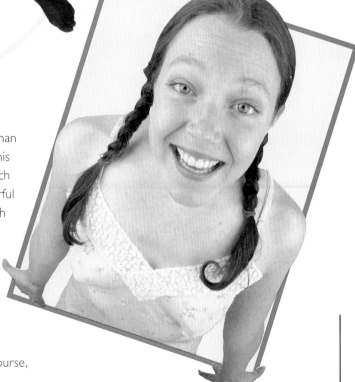

7
STUBBORNLY SINGLE

Spring seems to kick off the season. Everywhere there's the sudden appearance of cuddly couples. From movie theaters to restaurants, bookstores to clubs, no zone is safe. Fingers, hands, elbows, and arms entwine, two by two, in every nook and cranny one passes. Lips lock, knees quiver, and nimble limbs disappear in and out of clothing as once-modest singles become tawdry twosomes everywhere, it appears, except in your decidedly private, personal space. Stubborn singles are quick to spot this outbreak of "EE," or "Exponential Exhibitionism."

No one, it suddenly seems, is alone but . . . you! Teenage twosomes swoon over ice cream and clove cigarettes in the mall. Professional pairs share their lunch breaks like so many gray flannel and white linen salt and pepper shakers.

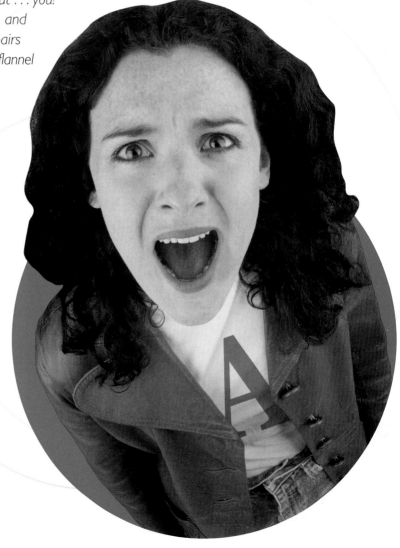

Choosing to remain single instead of spending time with a dolt just to have someone around to call a companion is a modern choice that, unfortunately, still comes complete with its share of outdated social stigma. It's fine when you're in your teens, playing the much-expected, oft-tolerated role of the lonely rebel. It's even okay during your twenties, when hopping in and out of reluctant relationships is acceptable, if not downright encouraged.

But late-twenty-to-early-thirty-somethings who dare to enter a restaurant, movie theater, bookstore, or concert hall alone on a Friday or Saturday night might just as well have a huge, scarlet "A" (for "A"-lone, that is) stitched onto their shirts.

Luckily, few seem to mind!

MY BLOODY VALENTINE, OR: MEET LOVE'S BIG LOSERS

Dread starts early. Stores stock their shelves in January with all things pink and red; one holiday has just passed and a new one looms, but worse than Christmas or New Year's, for it settles for nothing less than a pair.

Stubborn singles must endure the nauseous effects of second-hand billows of romance for not just one month, but two. The reminders seem everywhere: Ads for a candlelight dinner; e-commerce come-ons for everything from flowers and candy to decorated condoms. A two-seater bike with a single rider goes by. V-Day is coming, and you don't have a date.

BUZZ ON ASKS:

"What did you do for Valentine's Day?"

LOVE AT THE LAST MINUTE

"Last year I thought I'd get really romantic, right? Flowers, candlelight, candy, silk boxers, the whole route. Only problem was, my girlfriend chose that very morning to break up with me! Of course, I can't say that it actually came as a complete shock. Things had been getting a little stale lately, anyway, but, that's what Valentine's Day is for, right? Spice things up a little.

"Anyway, I wasn't letting all that hard work and effort go to waste. So, all day long at work I hung around the break room and vending machines trying to figure out what chicks were dateless for that evening. Turns out this babe in accounting I'd had a crush on for months was in the same boat I was. I asked her out, she accepted, and we had a blast. She thought it was really romantic and kept saying it was totally my ex-girlfriend's loss. We ended up dating for two years after that."

DINE AND DASH?

"My best friend and I have had a running 'Valentine's date' for the last five years. Dinner, a movie, and then we'd grab a couple of ice cream cones on the way home and not bitch about calories the entire time. But last year she had finally gotten serious with this guy she really cared about so I was on my own. Before, I'd always sort of looked forward to our 'date' and therefore never really understood why so many of my friends, co-workers, and peers hated Valentine's Day so passionately. Now I do. I felt like a pariah! Since it was too late to find a date of my own, I went ahead with our date as planned, only minus my best friend. I saw a movie in an empty theater, then ate dinner alone in a crowded restaurant full of happy couples.

"Finally, I made it to our annual 'dessert destination' and I was really looking forward to eating an entire quadruple-scoop ice cream cone all by myself. But after three licks I looked up to see my best friend and her date walk in! The place was pretty crowded, so I managed to sprint into the bathroom and find an empty stall. I didn't know what else to do! I panicked and felt like a total loser. I waited half an hour and then came out, just so the waitress wouldn't think I'd dined and dashed on her. My friend and her date were gone, but the waitress was really mad. I told her I'd had an allergic reaction to the waffle cone I'd splurged on and had been in the bathroom throwing up the whole time. I don't think she believed me."

3 - 1 = FUN!

"The creep I'd been dating was too much of a chicken to ask me if his friend could 'tag along' on our Valentine's date last year. I wouldn't have minded, it wasn't like we were doing anything special anyway, but when my boyfriend just showed up with his buddy and no explanation, I felt it was my duty to pout. Naturally, my boyfriend's friend thought he had told me and apologized about fifteen times on the way to the restaurant. My boyfriend ended up getting really drunk and acting like a fool, flirting with the waitresses. I asked the manager to call him a taxi, and after he was gone his friend and I finished our 'date' by having coffee at a little diner down the street. It was totally deserted and we had the whole place to ourselves. It turns out we had a lot in common and really enjoyed each other's company. We didn't start dating or anything, but we've remained really good friends ever since. Plus, it was a great excuse to ditch my lousy boyfriend."

BOYFRIEND BAGGAGE

"I just happened to have started going out with this guy a week before Valentine's Day. He was a friend of a co-worker and we'd met in a group situation, hit it off, and had had only two 'dates' before Valentine's Day. Everything was going really well. He seemed like a nice guy, had a decent job, and took good care of himself. Our first two dates had been fun and easy-going. Even though we hadn't slept together yet, I was looking forward to our first time together and, naughtily, was hoping it would be

Your	Gets
— girlfriend of one year	a romantic dinner for two.
— boyfriend of one year	a second chance to make up for last year!
— girlfriend of one month	a dozen roses.
— boyfriend of one month	a dozen beers (i.e. a twelve-pack).
— girlfriend of one week	edible panties.
— boyfriend of one week	edible jockeys.
— girlfriend of one day	to see you sober.
— boyfriend of one day	to sleep in the wet spot.
— backup date	whatever the hell he/she wants!

"You have to kiss a lot of toads before you find a handsome prince."

— American Proverb

on Valentine's Day. Anyway, he stopped calling me about February 12th. Just stopped. I had no idea why and just sort of assumed he was playing it cool, making big Valentine's plans, etc. By the evening of the 13th, I was getting a little antsy.

"Now, I'm no shrinking violet, so I just picked up the phone and called him up. He answered himself and was all cool like, so I asked him what was up. That's when he freaked out. It turns out he'd overheard me talking with a few of my girlfriends about how much I loved Valentine's Day, which was true. I know a lot of ladies hate it, but I've never taken it very seriously and have always managed to make a fun night out of it, no matter what I do. Anyway, he got all paranoid and assumed I'd only gone out with him to make sure I had a date for February 14th. He called me every name in the book and even accused me of 'using' him just for a Valentine's date and honestly believed I was going to dump him at midnight or something! Hmmm, can you say 'female issues'?"

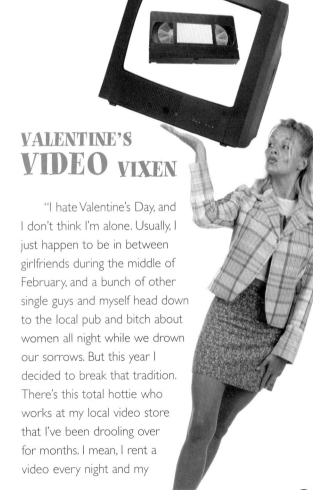

VALENTINE'S
VIDEO VIXEN

"I hate Valentine's Day, and I don't think I'm alone. Usually, I just happen to be in between girlfriends during the middle of February, and a bunch of other single guys and myself head down to the local pub and bitch about women all night while we drown our sorrows. But this year I decided to break that tradition. There's this total hottie who works at my local video store that I've been drooling over for months. I mean, I rent a video every night and my

VCR's been in the shop for years. That's how bad it is. So I wait until just before closing and then pop in to rent a video. The place is dead because everyone in the world is out on a date and I mope around the store for ten minutes looking as pathetic as possible.

"She doesn't seem in any rush to close up, so I assume she doesn't have a date either. I rent the biggest chick-flick I can find, and put it on top of this box of chocolates I've brought in for her as I head up to the counter. She smiles, grabs the video, and rings it up, then looks at the box funny before telling me that she 'doesn't sell that kind of candy here.' I tell her that it's a gift for her, and I'd love it if she'd come back to my place and enjoy it with the video, my treat. She hesitates for a minute and I'm sure some stud is outside waiting for her to get off work or something so they can spend the most romantic night of their lives together.

"But she finally says she's not quite comfortable with going back to my place on a first date. Yeah, right, I can take a hint. But then she shocks me by saying that we could use the VCR in the break room. We had a blast, made a real date for the next weekend and really hit it off. I've been getting free videos ever since."

ROLE REVERSAL

"I consider myself pretty romantic, but I like to be subtle about it. You know, little notes in my girlfriend's lunch box, soul music, daisies on her doorstep for no reason, that kind of thing. Naturally, a greeting card holiday like Valentine's Day really irks me, because it's like one of those 'absolve all' masses they have in the Catholic church. You know, where total, venal sinners who haven't gone to church all year get to show up and be absolved of all their sins and start clean. Just like that.

"Well, guys who don't do anything romantic all year get to show up on Valentine's Day with one of those stupid heart-shaped boxes of candy that they probably picked up at a gas station on the way over and all is forgiven. As far as I'm concerned, let my girlfriend do something romantic for a change. Naturally, she doesn't always agree with this one, tiny, chauvinistic opinion of mine. However, after three years of Blockbuster nights and Chinese food, she finally cracked. I came home from work to find daisies on the stoop, Barry White on the CD player, beer in the fridge, and those corny conversation heart candies leading a path to the dining room where she had a romantic candlelight dinner waiting for me. I won't mention what we had for dessert."

But What About This Year?

Say what you will about Valentine's Day, but despite all of our grumbles, mumbles, and groans, most of us will at least attempt to find a date for "the big day." There appear to be two schools of thought when singles turn their attention toward Valentine's Day: **Find** a date and join the "fun," or **make** a date . . . to bolt the doors with a box of chocolate and a bubble bath or two!

This first option, of course, combines all that sucks about finding a decent date in the first place, and adds to it the additional pressure of finding a date on a deadline. This is, of course, a little like cramming for an exam, with no chance of passing. You've probably rushed into a date with someone you don't really know, like, or remotely even care about.

The second option also sucks, because you admit defeat in early January and spend an entire month planning a night that is basically the candle-lit, chocolate stained, bubble-bathed equivalent of straightening your sock drawer on prom night.

There are hybrids to the first two choices, of course. Modern singles are nothing if ingenious when it comes to avoiding the real issue that Valentine's Day is actually a celebration of romance and love.

There is always the "group" date, which, on first glance, seems to solve all the problems associated with Valentine's Day in one quick, easy solution. For one thing, it is, technically, a real, actual date. When Mom calls on February 10th to ask, knowingly, "Well, dear, what are

you doing for Valentine's Day this year?" you can, without having to go to confession that weekend, reply truthfully, "Going on a date."

Unfortunately, group dates tend to cluster unevenly toward one sex over the other. It is rare that such dates are ever rationed out in a boy-girl-boy-girl seating arrangement. (If they did, they would be called double, triple, or quadruple dates, after all.)

No, the most likely scenario is that six grumpy girls cluster around a booth in some restaurant across town while one or two unfortunate males keep having to use the "restroom." In reality, of course, they are on their cell phones trying desperately to line up something, anything, else to do that night.

When they do, naturally, it leaves the six ladies with plenty of ammunition aimed straight at the male persuasion, as coffee is poured and men are dissed relentlessly, endlessly, even as the rest of the restaurant fills with romantic couples by the busload.

This leads to yet another option, the "stag" night,

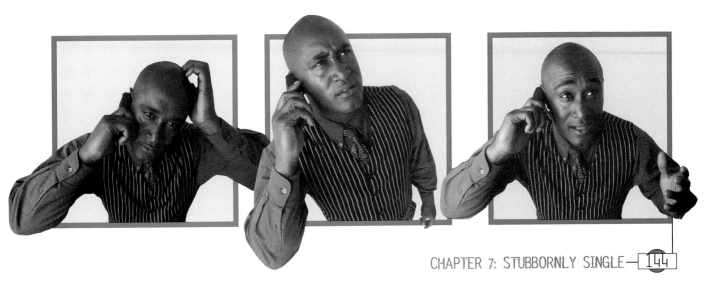

which is nearly exactly what has just happened above. However, in this instance, members of the opposite sex are eliminated from the equation altogether, leading, of course, straight to one long bitch session, where men and women equally enjoy a night of unbridled verbal passion, which appears to be the only kind they'll have this Valentine's Day!

Many singles opt for yet another hybrid option, the "blind Valentine's date." This is technically different from the very first option because, unlike those dates, this date is a one-time-only deal. A date that actually serves several purposes: Number one, it gets friends, mothers, relatives, sisters, brothers, as well as old boyfriends, off of your back so they won't feel sorry for you anymore. Or, at least, it gets these concerned souls off of your back until February 15th, when every single one of the above mentioned folks calls to see how your "big date" went and you tell them, in no uncertain terms, that it was a disaster.

The blind Valentine's date also serves to allow you to get caught up in the greeting card madness that sweeps the country during the second week of February. You too can stand in mobbed Hallmark lines and pay the price of most paperbacks for a simple greeting card just like everybody else. It may in reality suck just as badly as staying home and avoiding all of the fuss, but it won't seem like it because everyone else is right there with you.

There are toenails to paint, hair to get done, reservations to keep, a perky new shade of blood red lipstick to buy just for kicks, and then, of course, there's the date itself.

Oh, yeah, and there's the guy or girl. Which is, in all likelihood, the only *unpleasant* part of the blind Valentine's date. But if you play your cards right, you can always meet your date at the restaurant, grab a quick bite, wisely skipping the appetizer and after-dinner drink, and be home in time for the late show. When all is said and done, actually, not a bad way to spend an evening.

Although the chocolate and bubble bath route would have probably been more enjoyable, not to mention having cut out the middle man, or middle woman, entirely.

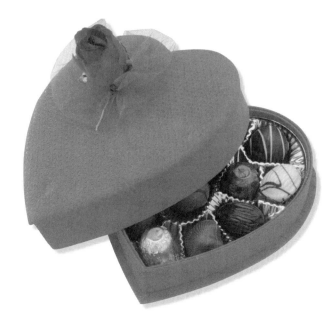

FOREVER FUTONS

Halfway between a sleeper sofa and a glorified milk crate, the futon is a relatively recent development in American furniture culture that has had serious repercussions on the modern dating scene. Essentially, the simple, inexpensive futon is a throwback to the days of Mary Tyler Moore's Hide-A-Bed-sleeping, loft-living, beret-throwing-in-the-middle-of-the-street, independent-modern-working-woman lifestyle.

Futons now make it possible for stubborn singles to not only have an extra room that used to hold a bed, but also they never have to make that non-existent bed ever again.

Today's modern singles can simply roll out of the futon in the morning, fold it back up, toss on some nattily accessorized throw pillows and go about their business, thus making every room a possible living room, study, or den, effectively eliminating, for all intents and purposes, the "bedroom" and all that might mean in a relationship.

Therefore, an unexpected benefit

TOP-5...

...Failed Futon Names

5.) The Squirminator
4.) More Cushion for the Pushin'
3.) *Video Camera Included
2.) The Iron Maiden
1.) The Casting Couch

to the single, who might not want to stay so forever, has arisen from the futon option. Basically, it comes from that "safe" feeling one has from sitting on an innocent-sounding couch instead of on a more sinister-sounding bed.

"Whoever called it necking was a poor judge of anatomy."

– Groucho Marx

"Well," the innocent victim thinks, enjoying a glass of wine and admiring the throw pillows, "we're on a couch ... what can happen?" Yet when that couch is actually a mere flick of the wrist away from turning into a full-blown bed, the more appropriate question might be, "What *can't* happen?"

Therefore the futon, for either sex in this ambiguously aggressive age, has become an inexpensive yet effective trap set for unsuspecting dates across the country. "How so?" you ask.

Consider the following, typical scenario:

Prey: "Knock-Knock."
Predator: "Hey. Hello. How are you? Did you find the building okay?"

Prey: "Oh, yeah, sure. Your doorman's cool."
Predator: "Yeah, I told him to be on the lookout. Hey, you look great. Come on in. Why don't I take your coat?"
Prey: "Oh, well, okay. I thought we had early reservations, though."
Predator: "Yeah, yeah, we did. But it turned out to be such a nice sunset, I thought maybe we could have a drink or two here first. So, I changed the reservation for a little later. You're not mad are you?"
Prey: "Oh, no. Actually, now that you mention it, it is a pretty nice sunset. That's awfully romantic of you."
Predator: "And this new futon I bought is so light, I was able to turn it to face the sliding glass doors. Why don't you have a seat and we'll toast the beginning of a wonderful evening."
Prey: "Ahhhhhhh, how sweet."
Predator: "Here's your drink. I hope you don't mind, all I had was Absolut vodka. The tonic went flat, I guess I was so nervous about our date tonight, I forgot to get some fresh. So, I made you an Absolut and Absolut. I hope you don't mind. How does it taste?"
Prey: "Cough. Gag. Cough. Oh, just ... great. Wow, with these tears in my eyes, the sunset's even more beautiful. And, hey, you know, this couch is pretty comfortable."
Predator: "Au contraire. It's better than a couch, it's a futon."
Prey: "Well, what's the difference?"
Predator: "Here, let me freshen your drink, then I'll show you."

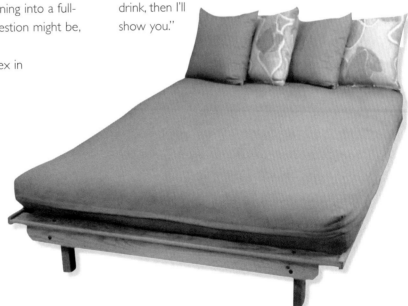

SINGLE BY DEFAULT

lovely lady you've been courting reveals his or her dark side? Feast your eyes on the following story to find out:

TATTOO YOU!

The misconception about stubborn singles is that they are, in fact, stubborn! (Other words include spoiled, picky, persnickety, and just plain pissed, but we won't go there.) Often this couldn't be further from the truth. Many singles are single by default. That is, they desperately want to be attached, involved, and even married. However, they're just not willing to be attached, involved, or married to someone they can't stand!

In fact, many singles try quite hard to find a suitable suitor. Sometimes, they even succeed and move on from the dreaded stubbornly single set to that of the comfortably coupled. Yet just as often their attempts fall flat on their face, through no fault of their own. Come on, you've been there:

The guy seemed great. No bad habits (you watched), no bad hygiene (you smelled), no hidden weapons (you snooped), and no criminal background (you checked). Then, on your fourth date, he asks you to tie him up, pour mint jelly on his head, and call him "Sylvia" while his favorite episode of *Star Trek* whines away in the VCR.

Or perhaps she came off as the perfect debutante. (At first.) Pretty, refined, genteel, and well-mannered. Her car was clean, her bookshelf filled with intelligent tomes, and there was none of that eye-twitching that was the sure tip-off as to her psychosis. So was it anything less than a bona fide shocker when, in the throes of passion late one night, she kept calling you "Daddy." (And not in a good way, either.)

After all, today's limited dating scene of movies, concerts, restaurants, and clubs doesn't offer much in the way of quiet conversation and the even more important lost art of observation. It's way too easy for the odd psycho or psychette to slip in under your finely tuned whacko radar.

So what happens when the perfect gentleman or

"What a fantastic night!" you think to yourself as you coyly drive him back to your place, despite the fact that he met you at the restaurant and you'll have to drive him back again to get his car later. As in—the next morning. At the moment, however, an early morning drive is the least of your worries. In fact, you have no worries at all.

Dinner was grand, expensive, exquisite, extra-long and—on him. He pulled out your chair, opened doors, ordered for you (after actually asking what you wanted), and hung on your every word.

As the manager of your local video store chain, you'd always considered him a bit of a nerd. Especially when dressed in his prepster tie, stiff Oxford shirt, and goofy blue "Videorama" apron. Yet slowly, over time, as he commented on your nightly rentals and even suggested some that had eventually turned out to be some of your favorite movies of all time, your sentiment changed. There was more to this man (-ager) than met the eye.

When he finally asked you out, after covertly expunging several days worth of late fees as a nifty little icebreaker, you said "yes" with only a mild case of hesitation. Now, after dinner, drinks, and an evening spent pouring out your soul, you were preparing for something you hadn't experienced in months (okay, years): a one-night stand.

You'd decided as much on the way home, in between the Dunkin' Donuts and the Exxon station, when your favorite romantic song came on the car stereo and, instead of turning it down like your last six dates would have, video boy had actually turned it up a notch and listened quietly while you drove.

Now he was back at the stereo, only this time it was located in your third floor apartment living room and tuned to the sexy soul station while you poured the wine and took off your shoes, two major signs of body language he could hardly escape noticing. And, which he didn't. Unhanding you of your wineglass, he kissed you gently even as your fingers reached to undo his tie and unbutton his shirt.

"Wow," you exclaimed by the time you'd reached the third button. "What have we here?"

"Oh," he stammered, nearly blushing. "That's just a little tattoo I got back in college. Just ignore it. Unless," he added hopefully, "it turns you on."

"A tattoo?" you ask, unbuttoning further to reveal a vibrant skin mosaic of reds and blues, yellows and oranges. "How exciting? What is it? A little heart? A tiny butterfly? Come on, let's see."

As you explore the expanse of his smooth, hairless chest, goosebumps, and not the good kind, score your half-naked flesh. (How quickly a turn-on can turn into a turn-off!) While he smiles proudly as you admire what he undoubtedly considers a masculine masterpiece, you try not to show your horror and distaste.

Had he stopped with the expertly coiled snake, which wound tightly around his left nipple, you might have had quite a different reaction. The implicit danger, fear, and excitement of a tattoo, one tattoo anyway, was a definite turn-on. What would your mom think? Your friends? How would it look gazing out from a clean, white tank top?

What would it taste like? Etc.

Unfortunately, your video store manager/ink junkie had gone hog wild with his tattoo review. The snake gave way to a soaring eagle, which jutted across a setting sun. Clouds rose to just below his Adam's apple (no wonder he always wore a stiff shirt and tight tie) and raging rapids extended to his belly button and, you were quite certain, far beyond.

Gingerly removing his shirt, for curiosity's sake only, of course, you revealed the pièce de résistance on his back: a patchwork of broad bands and stripes forming a frightening face that stretched from video boy's butt-crack to his buzz-cut!

On his arms were further tales expressed in pictures: a spider trapping a fly, a dolphin basking in the sea, and others too numerous, and nauseating, to mention.

"Wow," you say, handing him his shirt back unceremoniously, even as you back toward the door. "You're quite a piece of work."

"Art," he corrects you, rather firmly. "You mean I'm quite a piece of art."

"Hey," you counter, whisking open the door. "I was going to say 'quite a piece of crap,' but then I remembered I was a lady. Hit the road, Tattoo Boy."

His face crumbling, he stammers "W-w-w-why?" on his way out the door,

"Let's just say I'm afraid to find out where your 'babbling brook' dries up," you explain, eager to run to the phone and win this week's version of your long-standing 'worst date of the week' bet with the girls from the office.

"Shoot," you think, turning all three locks and arming the security system after he's gone. "Now I've got to find a new video store."

"THAT'S RIGHT, TABLE FOR ONE..."

HE SAID

It has finally gotten to *that* point: Franklin is a "regular." Like the old woman in the corner who keeps blowing out her candle and then re-lighting it, or the retired businessman who always comes to dinner in a three-piece suit, Franklin has his very own table, not to mention a waitress who simply looks at him kindly and says, "The regular?"

Her name is Marge and she is a feisty old Italian broad with hair as dark as the soles of his shoes and more energy than a college freshman. She smiles when she sees him come in on a Friday or Saturday night, just before frowning and giving him "the lecture."

"The lecture" is as familiar to Franklin as "the regular" is to Marge, and it's quite rare for her to dish up one without the other.

"Listen, kid," says Marge, a cup of coffee in one hand, the unnecessary menu in her other, "It's not natural for a young guy like you to come in here every weekend and sit alone. Good looking kid like you oughtta be out with a pretty lady on his arm, doing up the town. Not grumbling over your coffee and pie with the likes of me."

Franklin always shrugs and stirs his coffee several times before replying, "When I get a date, Marge, you'll be the first to know."

Marge always laughs before deteriorating into a coughing fit on her way back to the grimy kitchen where she spends six nights a week. Like Marge says, Franklin is a young, good looking guy who has, at twenty-eight, simply grown tired of faking his way through boring blind dates, failed fix-ups by well-intentioned friends, and basically any other kind of date where he isn't wowed by the girl in the first five minutes.

He wants to feel passion, lust, or at least a mild case of passing interest in the girl sitting across from him and, failing that, he would rather just sit alone at this point in his life.

And so, until something better comes along, he is content to dine alone and have Marge, a sixty-three-year-old waitress, be his stand-in date most weekends out of the month.

Of course, by now he's gotten spoiled by Marge's easy patter and the fact that she brings him coffee and pie without his even having to ask for them. Can any girl match up to such high expectations anymore?

SHE SAID

Olivia used to dread going anywhere alone. Oh, sure, a trip to the corner store for a carton of milk in case of emergencies was fine, but any place else and she required one of her legion of friends to accompany her. Slowly, however, over time, space, and the ravages of "old" age (i. e. her late twenties), Olivia's friends either moved away, got engaged, tied the knot, or were otherwise involved with significant others.

Therefore, if Olivia was to do anything at all other than sit on her couch and watch the world go by, she had to face up to the fact that, sometimes, she would have to venture out alone. Gulp. Big Gulp!

Naturally, this was difficult at first. So Olivia took baby steps. She started with a coffee shop. You know, a scone and a cappuccino on the way home from work. Nothing odd for an almost-thirty-something single girl to do on a Tuesday night. Right? Of course, so that none of her friends, co-workers, distant relatives, or neighbors would see her and think her the most pathetic thing on the planet, she drove over seven miles to a quaint little coffee shop clear on the other side of town.

And, once she looked out from behind the bulky newspaper she'd brought along as camouflage, she noticed something: she wasn't the only one alone. Not by a long shot. There were single girls. And single guys. Single women. And single men. They seemed happy, content, relaxed, and unfazed that there was no one taking up the barstool, easy

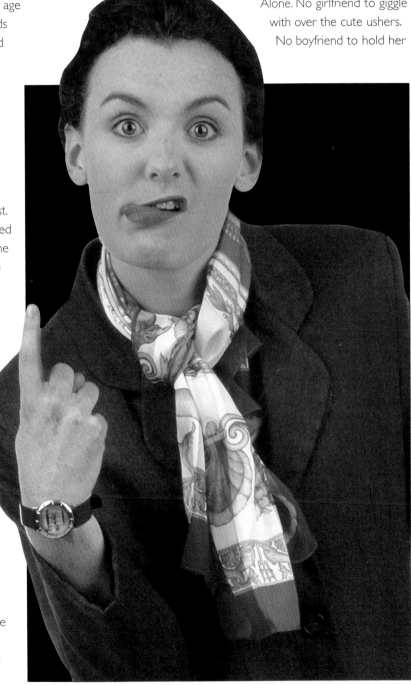

chair, or crumpled sofa next to them. Of course, it could have been all the caffeine they were sucking down, but Olivia thought it might be something more than that.

Since things went so smoothly at the coffee shop, Olivia figured it was time for the next step: a movie. Alone. No girlfriend to giggle with over the cute ushers. No boyfriend to hold her popcorn while she arranged her skirt. No "nothing" but herself and a single, lone, barren ticket-for-one to the latest special effects-laden, sci-fi cinematic romp through outer space. (Hey, it wasn't the movie that was important, it was the fact that she was there by herself.)

Again, things went without a hitch. No one she knew saw her to take pity on her as she wallowed in popcorn, aliens, and—self-pity. Of course, this could have been because she went to the multi-cineplex three counties over, but, nonetheless, she went. That was what mattered.

Finally, her crash course in "all alone alienation" complete, she took the biggest step of all: the dreaded table for one! At a local restaurant, no less. (After all, it was no fun driving for fifty miles all alone just so she could sit in a restaurant all alone before getting in the car to drive another fifty miles back—all alone!)

"I think, therefore I'm single."

– Female philosopher

Olivia went on a Saturday. No more baby steps for her. Feeling like she had been "outed," she wasn't ashamed of what was perfectly acceptable behavior. Sure, she was almost thirty and still single. Sure, it was a Saturday night and all of her friends were either out on dates or snuggled up next to their lovers enjoying a good video night. Sure, she would have rather had a chummy companion of the opposite sex to sit across from. But she wasn't going to ask out some boring schlep from work just so she'd have someone, anyone, to sit across from on date night.

Come to think of it, Olivia would rather be alone than spend another lousy date making bad conversation, listening to bad jokes, and, in general, having a *really* bad time. And so she went to the little vegetarian restaurant around the corner at 8 p.m., prime time, on Saturday, date night. She didn't blush. She didn't cringe. She didn't fumble as she asked for, gulp, a table for one. She didn't even squeal and run for home when the teenage hostess with the carrot-colored hair and numerous nose rings informed her there was a twenty-minute wait.

She simply nodded, grabbed a glass of wine at the tiny bar, and stood around listening to the faintly Moroccan music being piped in over the Muzak. She watched couples sit at other tables. She watched waiters carry trays laden with bean curd, tofu patties, and soy soup. She even watched her reflection in the Zima mirror behind the bar and smiled.

She was doing it. Eating alone. Dining unattached. She. Olivia. And it felt good. It felt right. For now, anyway.

"Olivia?" shouted the carrot-topped hostess. "Table for one? We're ready for you now."

Olivia finished her wine. Set it down on the bar. Smiled. Held her head up high. And followed the hostess. No one gasped. No one fainted. No one even turned a head.

Who knows? In this crazy, funky, quirky, awkward world of modern dating, maybe they had all asked for a "table for one" for themselves once or twice in the past. Maybe even more times than that.

TOP-5 Best Places to Go if You Want to be Alone

5.) The beach at night.
4.) A walk in the rain.
3.) A campus library on Saturday night.
2.) A museum.
1.) A Woody Allen movie.

5

TOP-5 Best Places to Meet Someone

5.) A wedding.
4.) At work.
3.) A campus library on Wednesday afternoon.
2.) The gym.
1.) The Laundromat. (Bring clean underwear!)

CHAPTER 7: STUBBORNLY SINGLE

"ALWAYS A BRIDESMAID" VS. "FOREVER A GROOMSMAN"

SHE SAID

Missy was almost thirty and had nearly as many bridesmaid's gowns and hideous pairs of shoes in the closet of her expensive one-bedroom apartment as she had birthdays. They ranged in color and shade from lemon chiffon to lime green Jell-O, and not one of them had been suitable for use at any occasion other than the wedding for which they were purchased. She'd considered trundling them all off to a local consignment store, but then thought better of it. If she only waited another thirty years, she'd have enough inventory to open her own used bridesmaid dress shop!

For the last ten years she'd watched countless friends, sisters, nieces, and acquaintances drive off, hand in hand with the one she loved, while Missy herself stood in front of the reception hall picking rice out of her hair and holding back the tears.

It was simply not fair. Half of the weddings she'd been invited to were in honor of hags who looked more like Frankenstein than his bride, yet still, by hook or by crook, they had managed to walk dreamily into the sunset with dentists or lawyers, podiatrists or college professors. Meanwhile, Missy continued through a seemingly endless procession of blind dates, bad dates, and no dates at all.

Missy realized that she was no Miss America, but she was twice as pretty as 75 percent of the brides she'd helped give away, and she marveled at how they did it.

As far as Missy could see, they possessed no secret charms, or even very obvious charms, for that matter. In fact, to a girl, they were decidedly less smart, less charming, less witty, less funny, and less discerning than Missy was herself. Yet they were living happily ever after while Missy continued looking for Mr. Goodbar.

And so, on yet another Saturday morning, she sat on the edge of her bed, milk chocolate stockings covering her legs and a hideous cream dress with brass buttons hanging over the bathroom mirror, her latest installment in the never-ending story of life as a bridal fashion victim. Soon she would be chewing on the inevitable rubber meatballs and washing them down with cheap champagne while yet another coworker strolled off into the sunset with that bald guy from accounting. She sighed, straightened her leopard skin scarf, and slipped into her thirty-first bridesmaid dress.

HE SAID

Across town, Felix tried in vain to fit into the tuxedo he'd long since purchased to avoid the hassle of renting one each time one of his friends, coworkers, brothers, cousins, or nephews tied the knot. It had fit just fine three years ago when he'd had the brainstorm to buy it, but nearly eighteen wedding receptions later, his spare tire was making it almost impossible for him to slide into his tuxedo pants, which he'd already had taken out twice.

"Sometimes I wonder if men and women really suit each other. Perhaps they should live next door and just visit now and then."

— Katharine Hepburn

Eventually he left the top button undone and covered it with the hideous caramel colored cummerbund provided by the groom. Unless he extended himself too far during the inevitable chicken dance, no one would be any the wiser. Walking through a mist of the good cologne he set aside for just such occasions (halfway gone now), he stared out of the sliding glass doors of his one-bedroom apartment and watched children at play in the park across the street.

It was a glorious Saturday, perfect for anything but getting married, at least as far as Felix was concerned. Despite his luxuriously casual bachelor pad, his big screen TV, and his dirty underwear, Felix was growing tired of being a groomsman and watching the same old schleps marry the same tired hags year after year.

It simply wasn't fair. Felix had long since sewn the last of his wild oats and had grown

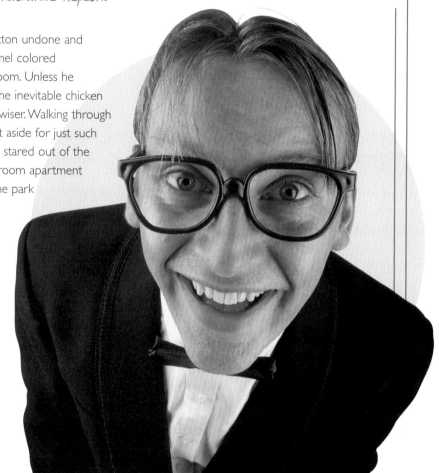

tired of the one-night stands and hungover mornings offered to him by the supposedly happening club scene. He'd had five long-term girlfriends in the last six years, yet when the appropriate time to pop the question eventually rolled around, he simply couldn't see himself spending the rest of his life with her, or her or her or her or even her.

And so he would break up, or, worse, act rudely or casually or slovenly enough to force *her* to break up with him. At least he felt less guilty that way, for a while anyway. And now, here he was, growing out of his secondhand tux and getting ready to attend yet another wedding where he would be forced to stand in line with another group of bachelors watching a mutual friend with less hair and worse teeth get married.

He drove his car to the church, applied his laughably beige boutonniere, and waited in line to help seat the guests.

THEY SAID

Missy dried the tears out of the happy bride's eyes even as she rolled her own in amazement. What did *she* have to cry about? Missy was the one who should be crying. Still, she tried to be cheerful and supportive for her friend, even as a chubby guy named Felix walked her up the aisle, muttering something under his breath the entire time.

"Excuse me?" she whispered halfway down the aisle.

"Oh, nothing," he said, seemingly surprised that he had been speaking aloud. "I was just commenting on the groom's back hair, which seems to be overflowing his tuxedo collar as we speak."

Missy brought the boringly beige bouquet in her hands up to her face to stifle a snort. "Try the bulging red boil on the bride's neck," she caught herself saying as Felix chuckled into his bow tie.

They reached the altar far too soon, but not quick enough to keep Felix from making a "date" for after the wedding pictures to meet at the bar for a drink.

For the first time all day, Missy wondered what a wedding gown would look like hanging in her closet next to all of those horrible shades of chewy cherry, orangutan orange, and lemon yellow.

For the first time all day, Felix was glad he already owned a tuxedo. Now, if he could just find a way to button his pants before his own wedding.

TOP-5...

...Tips for Attending a Wedding Alone

5.) Bring a "cool" dress to change into for the reception.
4.) Have an overnight bag in the trunk of your car, just in case.
3.) To avoid bad decisions, drink half as much as everybody else.
2.) Avoid catching the bouquet.
1.) Skip the chicken dance. (Nobody worth dating is on the dance floor anyway.)

8

MATRIMONY MATTERS

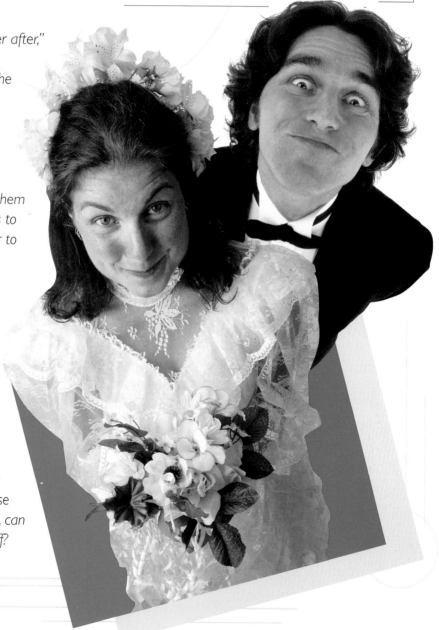

F ar from living "happily ever after," however, the stubbornly single's conjugal counterparts, the "modern marrieds," face their own battles in bliss-world. Sure, it may seem like they've got the world by the tail: A partner to cuddle with on chilly winter evenings. A better half to help them through the rocky times life has to offer. A hand to hold. A shoulder to cry on. A "happily ever after" to share. Forever.

But finding Mr. or Mrs. Right is only the half of it.

From perspiring over proposals to wondering where to register, young couples face a myriad of marital misgivings. And that's before the bachelor and bachelorette parties, where all kinds of problems can suddenly "arise," so to speak. But for those who make it through all of that, can a "happy honeymoon" be far off?

INSTITUTIONALIZED: THE HISTORY OF MARRIAGE

Throughout history, the institution of marriage was seen as just that: an institution. (Not unlike public schools, sanitariums, or prisons.) While sweaty palms, thumping hearts, and those lovable warm fuzzy feelings were nice, they were by no means a necessity for the bottom line: marriage was a legal agreement between two consenting adults. Period. End of story.

These ancient societies needed a secure environment for the perpetuation of the species, not to mention a strict system of rules to handle the granting of property rights. Accordingly, the sanctity of marriage "tied the knot" for both of these necessities. Love was simply the stuff of heroic legends, campfire stories, and fairy tales.

For example, an ancient Hebrew law actually required a man to become the husband of his recently deceased brother's widow. (Talk about, "till death do us part!") Naturally, this was to keep the family name intact and protect any and all rights to property. But, come on. Where's the love fellas? In this case, as in so many others throughout history, it was the woman who got the short end of the matrimonial stick.

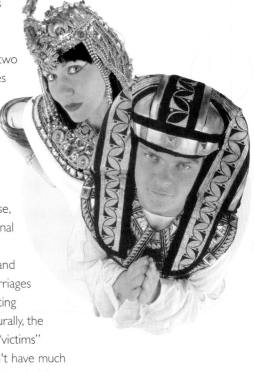

Different periods of time and even different cultures had very different histories when it came to women. Ancient Egypt, for example, gave women equal rights. In theory, anyway. But, as is the case with most theories, it wasn't always practiced. Medieval women had two responsibilities in life: one to religion and one to marriage. Enjoy!

Of course, many traditional cultures just went ahead and arranged marriages for unsuspecting couples. Naturally, the unfortunate "victims" involved didn't have much to say about the decision:

TYPES OF MARRIAGE

- **Polygamy:** one man, several wives or one woman, several husbands

- **Polygyny:** one man, several wives

- **Polyandry:** one woman, several husbands

- **Endogamy:** requirement to marry someone who belongs to his or her own group

- **Exogamy:** people have to marry someone from another area

- **Bigamy:** the crime of entering into a second marriage while the first is still in effect

- **Common-law marriage:** couple legally considered married depending on length of time together

- **Monogamy:** one man, one wife

MARITAL STATUS OF PEOPLE 18 YEARS AND OLDER, BY SEX

	MALE	FEMALE
MARRIED, SPOUSE PRESENT...	58 %	54 %
MARRIED, SPOUSE ABSENT	3 %	4 %
WIDOWED	3%	11 %
DIVORCED	9 %	11 %
NEVER MARRIED ...	27 %	20 %

"Congratulations, son," a resourceful father might say to his bargaining chip. "The village matchmaker and I have been hard at work finding you a perfect bride and we finally did. You are going to be the lucky husband of Esmeralda, the butcher's daughter!"

"Esmeralda!" the luckless son might gasp. "You mean that ugly girl with the horrible boil on her chin who shouts profanities at passersby as she sprawls across the town in her hair dress? But father, whatever for?"

"Didn't you hear me?" the impatient father might scold, eagerly carving wedding invitations into rock. "She's the butcher's daughter. Free meat for life, son. Free meat! No more gruel and goat milk for your mother and me. And, of course, you won't just be gaining a wife. Think of all those interesting new words she can teach you!"

It was the rare couple indeed who actually got married because they were in love.

Some marriages were actually issued by royal decree. As in, "Your hand in marriage, or your head in this basket." Others involved a dowry. As in, "Do you take this flock of sheep, gaggle of geese, herd of oxen and, oh yeah, this woman to be your lawfully wedded wife?"

At the other end of the gift-giving scale, some marriages required what was known as a "bride price." As in, "Dear sir, my honorable son, not to mention his extensive holdings, future earning potential, and diversified (live) stock portfolio, requests your daughter's hand in marriage."

Few of these misfit marriages involved any sort of casual courtship or dating, but most definitely had traditions. One almost universal tradition was that of the engagement ring. This custom can actually be traced back to the early Romans. Many historians assert that ancient cultures believed that the circular nature of the ring represented a new concept in time: eternity. Accordingly, the wearing of a wedding ring symbolized a union, not to mention a legal, binding, and business relationship, that was to last forever.

The notion of marriage as a covenant between a man and a woman and not just a contract between two legal entities can be traced back to that cuddly old romantic St. Paul, who compared the relationship of a husband and wife to that of Christ and his church.

Joseph Campbell, the world-renowned myth man, stated that the twelfth century troubadours were the first ones who thought of love in the compassionately cuddly way we do today. Naturally, this wellspring of romance, puppy love, and hot, monkey lovin' meant a rash of marriages taking place without witnesses, rice, or ceremonies throughout the 1500s. As a result, The Council of Trent decreed that marriages should be celebrated in the presence of a priest and at least two witnesses. (Was the advent of the marriage certificate far off?)

Years later, the Puritans referred to marriage as "the most blessed of relationships." They hypothesized that every day in a marriage was an opportunity to love, as well as a chance to forgive. (This from those warm and fuzzy folks who also brought you stockades.)

Throughout the nineteenth and twentieth centuries, of course, marriage was considered the ultimate goal for normal, healthy couples to engage in before, say, the age of nineteen or twenty. There was a little handholding, some discreet smooching, and, at even the faintest stirrings of that so-called thing called love, a proposal was struck, invitations were sent, and before you knew it you had a husband, one of those newfangled iceboxes, and three kids.

Slowly over the course of the 1900s, however, the institution of marriage evolved into a more personal decision. Sure, most women in the '40s and '50s thought they had the world by the tail as long as they were holding on to it with a hand bearing a wedding ring. But the sexual revolution of the '60s, not to mention the cancellation of those stereotypical sitcoms Leave It to Beaver and Ozzie and Harriet, gave women the freedom, independence, and confidence to hold out for something a little bit better. Whether that was marriage or not was, finally, up to them.

Today, of course, marriage is a personal decision of the highest order. Young couples, interracial couples, old couples, divorced couples, same sex couples, and transcontinental couples all enjoy the freedom to marry, or not marry, at will. In fact, to avoid becoming

an inevitable part of that pesky divorce rate, currently hovering at around 50 percent, many of today's modern singles are deciding to wait a while for Mr. or Miss Right. As for the future of that most romantic of institutions? Well, who can tell? We've all seen what kind of fun and frivolity can happen when you try to "Marry a Millionaire." But what about other televised marriages? Couples have been wed via the Internet. Is that the next big thing? Or how about mass marriages? Time will tell.

TOP-5 BENEFITS TO BEING MARRIED

5. Hey, ladies, you can never have enough copies of Sports Illustrated lying around.

4. "Date night" now consists of buying feminine products on the way home from Arby's.

3. Those tiny, unexpected pleasures: like setting fire to his old armchair.

2. One word: in-laws.

1. No more having to worry about those pesky orgasms.

INDECENT PROPOSALS

Like it or not, competition enters almost every aspect of American life. And, despite its once sacred status as one of life's most "breathless" moments, proposing to one's future spouse now carries a one-upmanship aspect usually reserved for the likes of professional wrestling. For instance, sappy shows such as the Lifetime Channel's *Portrait of a Wedding* (and its numerous rip-offs on other channels), bring modern, everyday couples (who just happen to look like the B-grade Hollywood actors they most certainly are) into the living rooms of millions of young singles who are secretly considering becoming un-singles themselves one day.

Of course, in an effort to make what should be a simple ceremony seem somehow more earth-shattering than agreeing to spend the rest of your life with the same person, such TV shows throw in a plethora of pre- and post-nuptial extravaganzas designed exclusively to make anyone but Donald Trump's daughter have "reception envy."

"I think men who have a pierced ear are better prepared for marriage. They've experienced pain and bought jewelry."

—Rita Rudner

Not content with ruining middle-class America's hopes and dreams of a perfect wedding, for who can compete with an all-expenses paid rehearsal dinner at Sandals resort in Jamaica or solid gold rose petals hefted down the aisle by a suspiciously steroid-shouldered flower "girl," marriage proposals themselves are taking a hit as well.

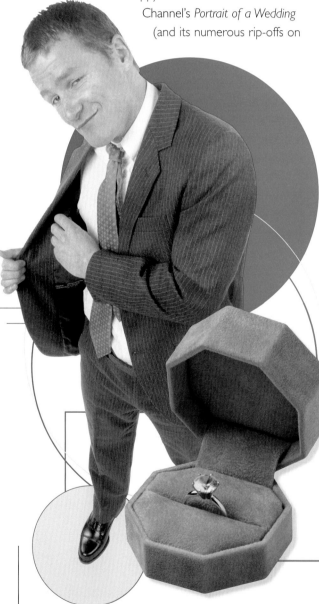

TOP-5 TIPS FOR POPPING THE QUESTION

5. Shave.
4. Have a camera ready.
3. Wear kneepads.
2. Bring tissue.
1. Don't forget the ring!

> "If it weren't for marriage, men would spend their lives thinking they had no faults at all."
>
> —Anonymous

A portion of most televised weddings necessarily begs the inevitable question, "All right, now for the important question: How did he propose?" The first installments of such shows were your average, run-of-the-mill, on bent knee, sweaty-palmed, cracking voiced proposals. But, like any other addictive drug that requires its user to take more and more just to feel "right," anxious audiences soon wanted "bigger and better" proposals to justify their viewing time.

Soon couples were not only outdoing each other, but outdoing the very bounds and limits of romantic decency as well, by heralding their self-promoting tales of rented hang-gliders and permanent tattoos, classified ads in *The New York Times* magazine, and prank phone calls to network news shows as ways of popping that all-important question.

For instance, there was the guy who froze the engagement ring inside of one very special ice cube and poured his intended a potentially potent "marriage martini." Or how about the guy who rented the biggest U-Haul he could find and paraded it down his girlfriend's street with a billboard size poster on its side that read: WILL 'U-HAUL' ME DOWN THE WEDDING AISLE?

Both of those pale in comparison, however, to the poor schmoe who had the bright idea of proposing to his girlfriend of two years by camping out along her path to work atop a four-story building with a roll-down banner at the ready! Little did he know his girlfriend and her roommate had switched cars for the morning. When he saw the telltale champagne gold Honda Accord pass by the building he was waiting atop

THE TRUTH ABOUT MARRIAGE

1 If you had to do it all over again, would you still marry your spouse?

- Yes 55%
- No 45%

2 Been around the block once or twice? Or maybe even farther? If you were to rate your relationship experience before trading rings, how far would you say you've traveled?

- 2-3 strolls around the neighborhood 45%
- This was my first time for everything 31%
- I've hit at least 3 continents 24%

3 How would you rank your libido since you first got hitched?

- Maximum overdrive: still got a strong engine ... 42%
- Low octane: it takes a while to get my motor running ... 36%
- Running on empty: there's not much left 22%

[Survey results courtesy of *Women.com*]

of, he let the banner roll: MARRY ME, ANGEL, AND WE'LL SCALE GREAT HEIGHTS!

Luckily, Angel's roommate had a cell phone and instructed the matrimonial message's intendee to get to the building jiffy quick before her boyfriend jumped off in despair.

So, heard any other good proposals lately?

BACHELOR PARTY: BUSTS OR BUST!

Throwing a truly great bachelor party is an act so uniquely passive-aggressive that it defies any kind of psychological explanation whatsoever. On the one hand, you're so happy that your best bud is finally getting married that you've decided to throw him the bash to end all bashes: plenty of porn, don't forget the strippers, naughty pastries, enough booze to pickle Pittsburgh, and plenty of disposable cameras to record it all for posterior, ehhr, posterity.

On the other hand, he'll be the only guy at the party who can't really enjoy it!

Still, those of us here at *Buzz On* who have actually been to just such a stag party (or two) and actually survived to tell about them, have put our heads together and come up with a surefire way to make the perfect bachelor party come off without a hitch. (Or an arrest, for that matter!)

DETAILS, DETAILS

Now, we all know boys will be boys. But does that mean you have to be bad boys? (Don't answer that.) Naturally, a bachelor party is a time for having fun away from the girls. Letting it all hang out and getting a little primitive. Still, there's no reason to be rude about it.

With a little simple planning, any bachelor party can rise above its singular stereotype to become a party worth remembering, and not one the groom would rather forget.

That's right, the groom. Remember him? It's his party, after all. So to make it memorable, follow these few helpful hints:

● Serve food. Yes, this seems like a no-brainer, but you'd be surprised how many bachelor party planners will spend hours on the Internet hunting down just the right ridiculous breast-shaped party hats and forget something as rudimentary as a simple bag of pretzels.

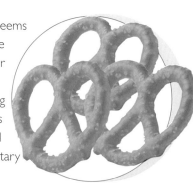

- Avoid hard liquor. Sure, sure. We know. Bummer, right? But a simple beer blast is much more likely to keep things orderly (as in, law and order-ly) in the long run. And, if you use bottles or cans, there's no need to invest in those pesky plastic cups! (Just make sure to have plenty of urinals handy.)

- Vary the guest list. Just because every one of the groomsmen is between the age of twenty-five and thirty doesn't mean you can't invite the bride and groom's fathers, brothers, uncles, cousins, etc. Sure, they may put a kibosh on your overnight trip to Tijuana to see that donkey act you've been hearing about, but you couldn't really find that missing passport anyway. (Besides, they're often the only ones sober enough at the end of the night to pay the bar tab!)

- Make plans for transportation. Most groups rent a bus or a van for the night, which is actually a good idea. Just don't get one that's too fancy, especially if you've got a bumpy ride home and a car full of drunk dudes seconds away from heaving up all those thoughtful munchies you so carefully planned on serving (see tip #1). After all, wall-to-wall carpet in a rent-a-van is a nice touch, but not when it costs you three hundred bucks to have it cleaned. (Or worse, you have to clean it yourself!)

TITILLATING TRADITION

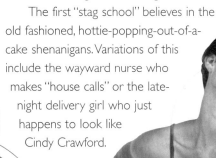

Ogling a stripper at a bachelor party is a titillating tradition that's been handed down for years and one that's become big business for topless clubs and exotic dancers across the country. Generally, there are two schools of thought concerning this "main event."

The first "stag school" believes in the old fashioned, hottie-popping-out-of-a-cake shenanigans. Variations of this include the wayward nurse who makes "house calls" or the late-night delivery girl who just happens to look like Cindy Crawford.

THE TOP-5 THINGS EVERY GUY SHOULD AVOID SAYING AFTER HIS BACHELOR PARTY

5 "Wow, when did strip clubs get rid of their 'hands off' policy?"

4 "I never knew $15,000 could go so far."

3 "Relax, sweetie. I sowed all my wild oats last night."

2 "Uhm, remember all those twenties we were saving for the honeymoon?"

1 "Boy, honey, I never knew breasts could get so big!"

Either way, in this scenario the main event takes place inside the home and that's the way they like it.

On the other hand, most of today's budding bachelors prefer to pile into a rented van and then proceed to hit every strip club in town. Naturally, there is little ceremony here to celebrate the groom's departure from single life. This is simply an excuse for eight to ten horny guys to get out for a night of bar tabs and debauchery.

So what's the be solution? Simple: Be yourself. Know your limits—and your libido. Be good. (Just not *too* good'

TANYA'S TALE

Man, I hate bachelor parties. I really do. Guys get so stupid at those things. It's like they check their brains at the door and so instead they take all their advice from between their legs. Plus, I work in a pretty small town, so a lot of times I'm dancing for guys I see every day at the grocery store or post office. Not that I'm embarrassed of what I do. I work hard for the money and I earn every cent. It's just that I lose so much respect for these stupid fools standing there in their argyle sweaters and deck shoes with a lei around their neck all laughing and grunting and making stupid gestures.

Just once I'd just like to bring a video camera in with me and show the tape to them the next day and see their expressions. I bet they wouldn't even believe it was really them if I did that. Still, bachelor parties can be pretty good money. I just need to move to a bigger town, that's all.

SINDERALLA'S STORY

In general, the guys I dance for are pretty sweet. But then, I'm a strictly freelance dancer, so I only make "house calls." You know, like out of the phone book. And the guys who call me tend to be the ones who are too scared to step foot into a topless bar in the first place. Most of them are tipsy, sure, but occasionally you get a bunch of Bible thumpers who are just going through the motions. Man, there's nothing worse.

I mean, I actually prefer it when the guys are drunk. At least then I don't feel like I'm being watched so closely. You know? I go in, do my stuff, pose for a couple of pictures with the groom, sign a couple of "autographs," maybe have a bite to eat, and I'm gone before things get too rowdy.

But non-drinkers, they're the worst. They watch every second of your act and don't make a bit of noise. Plus they're horrible tippers! It's just you and the stereo and a bunch of horny, but quiet, non-tipping guys. That's when I wish I drank!

A WATCHED POT NEVER BOILS

Ladies, we haven't forgotten about you. We know how frustrating it is to sit at home like the jilted school marm while your husband-to-be cavorts mere inches away from heavenly hotties with only a rainbow pastie separating him from good vs. evil. So don't!

Whoever said you had to sit home and let the boys have all the fun? Sure, since your sex is light years smarter than those goofy guys, you've planned ahead and had your bachelorette party a full week in advance of the wedding, just in case one of those Chippendales dancers got a little too close and gave you a black eye. (Wink, wink, nudge, nudge). So naturally you can't get anymore revenge than you've already had.

But that's still no reason to sit around the house alone watching the numbers on your digital clock blur and roll over. Why not get out of the house and have some fun of your own? Take in a double feature of chick-flicks you know he'll never want to accompany you to. Drown your sorrows by hitting every sushi bar from here to Poughkeepsie. (Just make sure you have a good seamstress if you choose this option!) Plan on having a slumber party with your bridesmaids and stay up all night playing truth or dare.

Either way, sitting at home and waiting for your fiancé to stumble through the door smelling of cigars and cheap perfume is no way to spend a bachelor party. Come to think of it, are you any good at jumping out of cakes?

BACHELORETTE
PARTY: SHE SAID!

While the typical bachelor party inevitably self-combusts into a veritable love fest of booze and broads, your average bachelorette party tends to rise above that lascivious level. Now, don't get us wrong. The ladies come to play just as hard as the guys do. They just do it with a little more style.

And, since we've already done it for the guys, we might as well help you ladies (like you really need it) plan the bachelorette party to end all bachelorette parties. (You do plan on ending your party, right?)

NAUGHTY NIBBLES

Of course, you can't have a great bachelorette party without great food. (What would Martha Stewart say?) And not just "food" food, either. We're talking about themed food. Dirty Dishes. Naughty Nibbles. Saucy Snacks. You know what we mean. Hot dogs. Wieners. Franks and beans. Buns. Meatballs. They'll all work as long as they're served with a wink and a smile.

Don't forget the drinks. Sure, it's up to each guest to choose her poison. But it's up to you to serve it up right. After all, what's a margarita on the rocks without ice cubes resembling male genitalia? But don't stop there. You can't serve a drink like that in any old Dixie cup. You've got to at least take a trip down to the local novelty store for a carton or two of Dicky Sippers. What's that? You've never heard of a Dicky Sipper? Then you're not living, missy. What bachelorette party would be complete without this six-inch, plastic, flesh colored hollow penis complete with a ten-inch straw?

And that's just the beginning. Today there's a whole division of catering services devoted to nothing but tasteless treats. From sheet cakes shaped like male torsos (complete with a condom candle) to anatomically correct lollipops, no bachelorette party would be complete without the best-selling "Penis Party Pack" from your local daring distributor!

DASTARDLY DECORATIONS

But it's not just caterers who are cashing in on the recent popularity of bachelorette parties. Interior decorators have their hands out as well. From pornographic place mats to dirty dishcloths, it only takes a few broad strokes of your party planner's passion to turn any old living room or den into the steamy sex palace it's about to become.

And don't forget the games. Who can resist a rousing drinking game of Pass Out or a whack or two at a penis-shaped piñata? Too much movement for your tastes? Why not try a simple game of pin the hard-on on the hunk? Too cheesy, huh? How about doodling with one of those pens that reveal a different kind of "ballpoint" whenever you turn them over? Or how about a rousing game of bridge with a dirty deck of cards? (Talk about a full house!)

Who knew the male member was so versatile?

FRESH FAVORS

But wait! Don't let your guests go home "unsatisfied!" Instead, send them packing with an assortment of genitalia goodies guaranteed to get them in gobs of trouble. For starters, we all know a simple three-by-five inch frame isn't exactly risque. But fill it with perky Polaroids of the stripper shenanigans to come, and it's sure to be one keepsake they treasure for a lifetime.

How about the latest issue of *Playgirl* for an added surprise under their seat cushion or paper plate? Although it may be hard to gain their attention for the rest of the night, at least you'll know they're enjoying your thoughtfulness. And while we're at it, why let the bride of honor have all the fun. Why not send your guests packing with a pair of edible panties to spice things up in their own home? They come in appealing flavors these days, from sparkling champagne to banana daiquiri, and they're guaranteed to spread the blush around. Not frisky enough? Try flavored condoms instead? But we're not done yet. Don't forget the reason you're all gathered together, to send off your best friend in style!

After all, it's not just pastries getting naughty these days. There's an entire assortment of presents out there. From pecker-shaped pacifiers to naughty fortune cookies, from the Big Boy shaped cake mold to the Bob-It Blow up Doll (handcuffs included) the world is at your disposal ladies. (Just remember to keep your receipt!)

TOP-10 THINGS YOUR FIANCÉ DOESN'T WANT TO HEAR AFTER YOUR BACHELORETTE PARTY

10 "Hey, you're the one who always says, 'honesty is the best policy.' "

9 "You know how I get after a couple of white Russians."

8 "I have no idea where that man's g-string came from."

7 "Remember when I said, 'size doesn't matter?' "

6 "Why, I always button my blouse like this!"

5 "Remember when I said 'cold feet was for wimps?' "

4 "If you must know, your mother brought the penis shaped eclairs!"

3 "Have you ever heard the term 'comparison shopping' before?"

2 "There's someone I think you should meet."

1 "Do you have room for an extra groomsman?"

THE MAIN EVENT

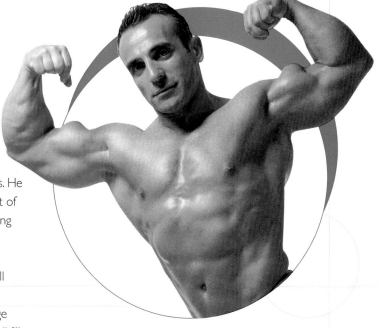

Naturally, all of this build up is in honor of one very special guest. You know the one. He usually shows up about halfway through the bachelorette party. This gives him just enough time to make sure you're all nice and inebriated so he's not "performing" to a bunch of stiff skirts, church ladies, and bad tippers. He won't be hard to recognize. Generally, he'll appear out of nowhere dressed in an ill-fitting and not very convincing police, delivery, or doctor's uniform. (Pick one.)

He will have a brilliant cover story: "Uh, there's been a complaint about the noise. Did someone call the cops?"

"Knock, knock. Did someone order an extra large with (wink, wink) sausage and (nudge, nudge) meatballs?"

"Pardon me ladies, but I'm a licensed physician. I heard someone here has a fever and needs my special love injection!"

Naturally, this cop, delivery guy, or doctor will just happen to be making an arrest, delivery, or house call at 10 p.m., not to mention carrying a boom box and a ratty backpack full of assorted oils, CDs, and business cards. Before you know it, this "surprise" guest will have rearranged your entire living room to resemble a cut-rate dance floor and "Everybody Dance Now" (how original) will be blasting through the house. Shortly thereafter, your detective, delivery boy, or doctor will disrobe with quickness and cavort around the room urging the bride-to-be to variously rub oil on, caress, or tip him.

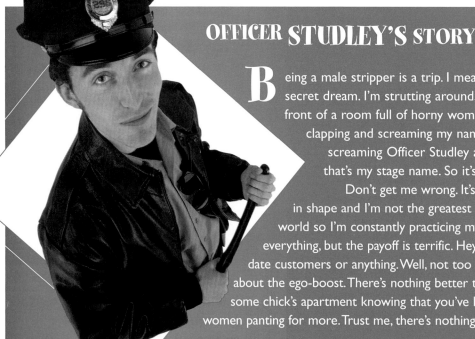

OFFICER STUDLEY'S STORY

Being a male stripper is a trip. I mean, it's every guy's secret dream. I'm strutting around, basically naked, in front of a room full of horny women who are all clapping and screaming my name. Okay, they're screaming Officer Studley at the moment, but that's my stage name. So it's just as good.

Don't get me wrong. It's hard work staying in shape and I'm not the greatest dancer in the world so I'm constantly practicing my moves and everything, but the payoff is terrific. Hey, I'm no slut. I don't date customers or anything. Well, not too often. I'm talking about the ego-boost. There's nothing better than walking out of some chick's apartment knowing that you've left a room full of women panting for more. Trust me, there's nothing like it.

Flash bulbs will track his every movement and, since the real guest of honor is being good tonight, he will hone in on the groom's mother-in-law, who's currently staring a hole into her shoes. Before long she will not only be dancing with him, but she'll have a hand full of oil, her wallet will be empty of singles (not to mention that five she'd been saving), and her pocketbook will be full of business cards!

Now, who says guys have all the fun?

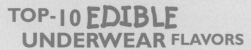

TOP-10 EDIBLE UNDERWEAR FLAVORS

10. **Passion Fruit**
9. **Strawberry Chocolate**
8. **Pink Champagne**
7. **Piña Colada**
6. **Cherry**
5. **Banana**
4. **Strawberry Champagne**
3. **Forbidden Fruit**
2. **Kiwi Strawberry**
1. **Mai Tai**

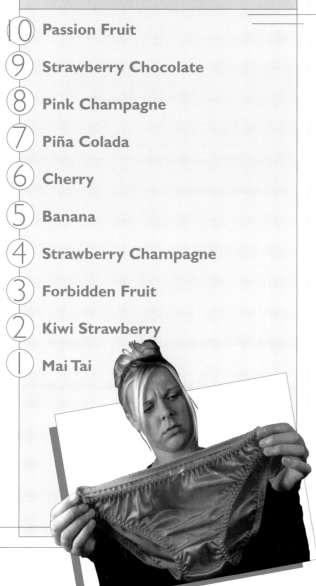

PETER THE PIZZA GUY'S PREDICAMENT

I don't know why, but male strippers don't get much press. Sure, everybody knows who the Chippendales dancers are, but the rest of us are just supposed to feel like sloppy seconds? I take my job very seriously and try and put on as good a show as possible. That's why I like bachelorette parties so much. I've talked to female strippers before, and they say there's a big difference between the way guys respond to them and the way girls respond to us.

For one thing, girls don't tend to drink as much as the guys do. Sure, the ladies will get a buzz on and scream out things that would make Howard Stern blush, but they're not falling all over the place like the guys are. And it seems like they appreciate a good performance more than the guys do. For most guys, a female stripper could do the moonwalk to accordion music and as long as she ended up naked they'd be happy.

But the girls are more challenging. They want to see a show, not just some guy's buns and a bulge. (Okay, they don't mind seeing that too.) That's why I get mad when people call me a stripper. I'm not just a stripper. I really am an exotic dancer. I give those women a show, and they appreciate it. Why do you think so many of them hand me their phone numbers afterward?

WEDDED BLISS(TERS!)

Okay, so you made it through the bachelorette party. You finally got over that nasty case of cold feet. You even had the "You do know what to do on your wedding night, dear?" talk with your Mom. Now all that's left to do is walk down that aisle (*for the rest of your life*), offer your own hand in marriage (*for the rest of your life*), and spend the *rest of your life* with that charming guy who you're quite sure will one day, eventually, learn to put the seat down. (After all, you have *the rest of your life* to train him!)

In order to make your day more memorable (as if committing yourself to the same man *for the rest of your life* isn't memorable enough), here are a few tips to help you make the most of the greatest day of (*the rest of*) your life:

EAT!

Hey, you're the one who's been dieting since he popped the question. Don't you think you're entitled to a Swedish meatball or two? After all, if you're like seventy-five percent of young couples today, you'll be paying for this wedding for the next, say, seventy-five years. Isn't that reason enough to chow down?

Go ahead. That's it. Wave good-bye to Uncle Harriet. Separate yourself from your new husband's a-little-too-enthusiastic younger brother. Strap a napkin around your beaded choker and chow down. Taste those asparagus fries. Enjoy those Portabello poppers. Swill that Brie fondue. Nosh those California rolls—hey, take it easy there, missy! Don't forget, you've still got that sexy negligee to fit into later tonight. (Save the grazing for your honeymoon!)

GREET

Sure, sure. It is *your* wedding. But part and parcel of throwing a wedding in the first place is meeting and greeting all those distant relatives who've traveled halfway across the globe to be there. Okay, so maybe you haven't gotten over the fact that Cousin Tommy liked to play doctor a little too much when you were kids. But is that any reason not to at least wave in his direction? (Considering the fact that he's been following you around since the ceremony ended?)

Likewise, it's essential that you make it a point to give the blue-haired senior citizen set their due. Anytime you see a cane, walker, or pair of nude thigh-highs pooled around age-spotted ankles, reel yourself in and stop on by. Don't diss your bridesmaids, either. Even though they're busy gettin' busy with the groomsmen, you never know when you'll need one of their shoulders to cry on later in life. (Not that you didn't marry the perfect man, that is.)

Don't forget, you never know who gave you what until after the wedding. So it helps to be kind to all until you're back from the honeymoon and you and your new hubby get a handle on who the family cheapskates, skinflints, and big spenders really are. So play along, smile for the drunken photographer with the bad toupee, and think of all that loot you'll get to inspect when you get back from your honeymoon. (Once you've slept for about seventy-two straight hours, that is!)

RETREAT

Don't forget to be good to the most important member of the bridal party: you! Take some time out for yourself. Sure, your face is tired from smiling and your hands are sore from shaking. Not to mention that corset around your waist is making it hard for you to breathe and your shoes (purchased one size smaller than usual) are pinching your toes into unrecognizable stumps. Grab a martini, hide it under your veil, and take a seat in the farthest stall from the door in the nearest ladies room.

Smoke a cigarette. Nosh some Jordan almonds. Nibble on some birdseed, for Pete's sake. Whatever it takes. Just remember that this is one of the biggest moments of your life. If you don't take time out to smell the roses, or in this case the Sani-flush, you'll miss the greatest moments of all. (Like when that witch from grade school, Susie Wannamaker, runs out of toilet paper in the next stall!)

COMPLETE

. . . your bridal duties. Okay, sure it's a drag. But those pictures have to be taken. The bouquet has to be thrown. The cake has to be delicately fed (or smashed) into each other's mouths. And, no matter how much you detest it, the inevitable rendition of "Y. M. C. A." has to be played.

When in doubt, smile, smile, smile. After all, with the plethora of TV shows like *Amazing Hidden Wedding Videos* and *Shocking Bridal Blunders* garnering higher and higher ratings every week, you never know when a covert corsage cam or Beta boutonniere is tracking your every move. (You don't want to win the "Bitchiest Bride of the Week" contest, do you?)

(BE) FLEET

. . . of foot, that is. When it's time to go, it's time to go. Period. Sure, everyone's having fun. There's singing. There's (chicken) dancing. There's sweating. There's eating. There's smiling. And all you've got to look forward to is a long drive to the airport with a hair full of rice and a lifetime of marital bliss with your new hubby.

But take heart. The DJ won't keep spinning "I Will Survive" and "My Funny Valentine" forever, you know. The chafing dishes will run out of Sterno, the bartenders will pack up their bottles and stir sticks, the caterers will scamper off with thirty pounds of peel 'n

eat shrimp, and it's been two full hours since Uncle Levi vomited. (So he's due any minute.)

No matter how much fun everyone (else) seems to be having, never forget that a wedding reception dissolves quickly after you're gone. (Or, at least, that's what your friends will tell you when you call from the honeymoon suite in Hawaii.) So hitch up your gown, close your eyes, wade through that sea of blinding birdseed, and don't look back.

(Married) life is calling. And you've decided to answer . . .

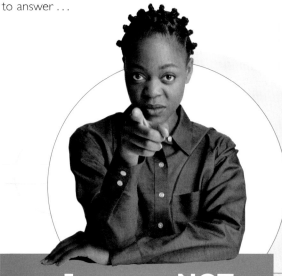

TOP-5 REASONS NOT TO VIDEOTAPE YOUR WEDDING

5 Two words: Instant replay.

4 Half of the bridal party would have to have their identities masked.

3 You tried that the first four times and it just didn't work out.

2 Court TV already owns the rights.

1 The Federal Witness Protection Program frowns on it.

HAPPY HONEYMOON:
FAIRY TALE OR URBAN LEGEND?

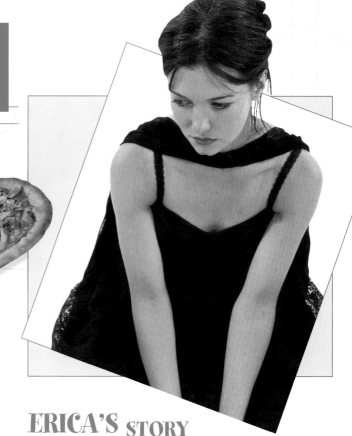

There are several "classic" scenarios that, in one form or another, repeatedly grace the amateurishly lit covers of XXX video boxes across the country. The pizza delivery boy meets the horny housewife is always a favorite. The prim schoolmarm who not so primly takes off her glasses and lets her hair down for the willing quarterback (or football team) is yet another.

Ever wonder why an average newlywed's hot and heavy honeymoon, which would seem to be a no-brainer to even the adult film industry, is not one such steamy scenario?

The answer is quite simple. There is literally no empirical data that has ever been compiled with which to write, direct, or film such a scene. Because, in a secret shared only by married couples themselves and often assisted by a "gag-order" signed in invisible ink on one's wedding certificate, the supposed postnuptial passion of a couple's hot and steamy wedding night is just another urban legend, like the gangs who kill people for flashing their high-beams and the killer who stalks the local lover's lane with a hook instead of a hand.

ERICA'S STORY

The resort was swank, remote, classy, and expensive. Of course, neither of them could afford it, but then, neither of their parents could have afforded the big wedding they'd just endured for the last seven hours either. The still happy couple figured, "Hey, if our parents just went into debt for us to get married, we might as well start the marriage in debt so they don't feel so bad."

FAVORITE HONEYMOON HOTSPOTS:

- Las Vegas
- Hawaii
- Niagara Falls
- Club Med
- Paris
- Cayman Islands
- Tahiti
- Saint Maarten
- Jamaica
- Walt Disney World
- Bahamas
- Costa Rica
- Bermuda
- St. Lucia
- Sandals Resorts
- Aruba
- U. S. Virgin Islands
- Anyplace else (as long as it's on a cruise!)

It had rained the whole way from the reception to the Miami hotel, where they were only staying for two nights before leaving for a ten-day cruise they could also not afford but had been looking forward to ever since she'd said, "I do!"

While Hampton frowned at the foggy windshield, Erica assured him that rain on your wedding day was actually good luck. "It gets all the bad stuff out of the way or something," she said as he smiled. They were married, and he was the happiest man in the world.

Erica had been nervous that morning. Not just "cold feet" nervous, but "run away and live in Tahiti for the rest of your life" nervous. She'd shown up late to the church for rehearsal the night before, and she'd seen that disappointed look in Hampton's eyes. She wasn't sure she could spend the rest of her life

YOUR PERSONAL "PLANNING A HONEYMOON" CHECKLIST:

- ✓ Use a travel agent to make your reservations.
- ✓ Use FedEx to get your tickets.
- ✓ Define the word "all-inclusive."
- ✓ Not enough room in your luggage? Skip the underwear.
- ✓ Make sure the hotel offers room service!

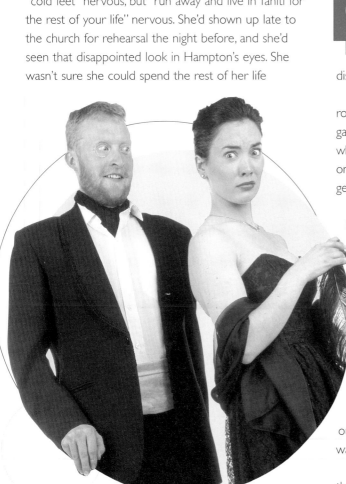

disappointing him.

She'd spent a restless night in her parents' guest room, until her mother saw her light still on at 2 a.m. and gave her a piece of bedtime advice, "Your heart said 'yes' when he proposed, but it's your brain talking now. No one ever found happiness listening to their brain. Now get some sleep, you've got a big day ahead of you."

She felt nauseous all morning, until her father clasped her arm gently and began leading her down the aisle. Hampton stood next to the priest, his smile beaming, his hands shaking, and a calm washed over her and she suddenly knew she'd made the right decision.

Now they were both exhausted, but married, and checking into the ridiculously snooty hotel where no one spoke English and everyone made you feel guilty that you noticed.

A British soccer team, in town for some game or another, admired Erica in her expensive "going away" outfit, a slim little cream number she'd picked out especially for those last few rice-throwing, waving-good-bye pictures at her reception.

To a man, they all said, "Hello" to her as they passed:

"Hello."

"Hello."

"Hello."

"Hello." And on and on it went. She blushed as Hampton returned with their room key. When he caught the end of the British "Hello" parade, he smiled broadly and said, "My new bride thanks you." The English blokes had a good laugh and congratulated him.

They left the bags in the car and walked across the street to a semi-famous restaurant where the dinner rush had just ended. Still, they sat at the bar and had a quiet drink to themselves before taking a cozy table for two overlooking the ocean.

Hampton, of course, proceeded to announce their marriage to everyone he could. The busboy. The maitre d'. The barmaid. The waitress. The regulars at the bar.

"We just got married," he'd say proudly, and she knew it wasn't just to get a free drink.

They chatted quietly over cocktails about who had or hadn't made a fool of themselves at the reception, and shared memories of the ceremony, the pictures, the family, and the friends.

They devoured mixed nuts, appetizers, and lobster, not having had a single moment at the reception to eat any of that wonderful food. Halfway through dinner Erica stooped to retrieve her napkin and half a bag of politically correct birdseed poured onto the floor. The happy couple laughed until they cried.

Erica rested her head on Hampton's shoulder on the way back to the hotel, stopping only for her overnight bag from the toilet paper and shaving cream-covered car. Every cell of her body screamed exhaustion, and she realized she hadn't slept more than four hours a night for the past week. Between second thoughts and worries about invitations and seating

TOP-10 ITEMS TO BRING ON YOUR HONEYMOON

10. Your driver's license. (In case you get carded!)

9. Your passport. (In case you get busted!)

8. Flavored condoms.

7. All that see-through lingerie you got at the bachelorette party.

6. Edible undies.

5. No-Doz.

4. Whipped cream.

3. Dollar bills for tips.

2. Any envelope you receive at your wedding reception (i.e. cash)!

1. It's a tie: Contraception vs. Film!

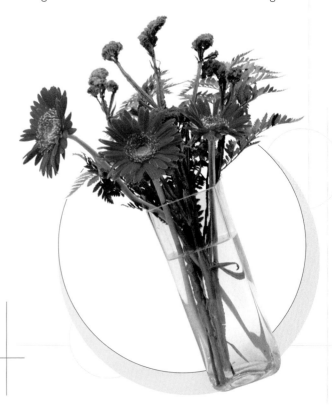

HONEYMOON HORROR: 30% DON'T DO THE DEED ON WEDDING NIGHT

How's this for a honeymoon horror—many newlyweds are just too exhausted to do the deed on the wedding night. That's according to a survey conducted by The Knot Web site, which reveals 30 percent of newlyweds admit they didn't have sex on their wedding night, and more than half say it was because they were just "too damn tired." Other matrimonial stats:

- 63 percent of couples became "born-again virgins" and abstained from sex before their weddings.
- 38 percent of couples kept themselves pure for at least a month before the big day, but 36% admit they only withheld from sex for one week before their wedding day.
- And, finally, 63 percent of brides admit their new hubby didn't carry them over the threshold on their wedding night.

arrangements, alterations and family altercations, champagne and wedding cake, she'd lived, breathed, and not-slept wedding plans.

Of course, Hampton had simply nodded and approved of every choice she made, and so was full of vim and vinegar in an elevator ride that would have made Madonna blush. She giggled and held the overnight bag to her side, knowing it concealed the sexy lingerie she'd received as a gag gift at her bachelorette party.

Little did her college friends know she'd envisioned Hampton's reaction the second she saw it.

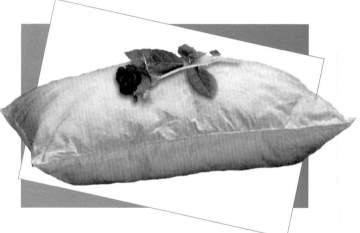

The honeymoon suite was overrated. The "Jacuzzi" tub was a rip-off and the remote control didn't work, but the happy couple didn't mind. Hampton placed a floral arrangement he'd managed to steal from the reception next to her side of the king size bed, and poured a nightcap from the bar. Erica slipped into her daring nightgown in the fully mirrored bathroom, realizing she'd probably never be so thin again after months and months of dieting to fit into her wedding gown.

Despite her anticipation, she yawned and slunk out of the bathroom door to Hampton's enthusiastic whistles and catcalls. He too had preparations, and disappeared into the busy bathroom with his shaving kit and a mischievous smile.

Erica propped herself up in bed alluringly, took one

last sip of Kahlua on the rocks, and promptly drifted into a dreamless sleep that would last the next seventeen hours.

She never saw the hilarious thong bikini underwear Hampton had also received as a gag gift at his bachelor party and had promised his best man he'd wear one time and one time only. She never saw him turn out the light by her bed, arrange the flowers gently one more time, kiss her on the forehead, which still bore the impression of her twelve-pound bridal tiara, or cover her up for the rest of the night.

She only saw him sitting there by the bed when she woke up at two in the afternoon the next day, patiently waiting for their honeymoon, and the rest of their life, to begin.

9

A GENERATION GROWS GROUCHY

They can't stay young forever, and as a young generation grows old, few of them are doing so as gracefully as they might have once imagined. With the individuality and uncompromising honesty that defines our particular generation, we limp forward with an unblinking eye and the same kind of questions every other generation has faced as it teeters toward the end of its thirties: "Hey, who let all these kids in here?"

As we find ourselves faced with expanding waistlines and diminishing hairlines, our generation grows decidedly "grouchy." No one wants to be called "sir" or "ma'am," but as the onslaught of time marches on, the possibility of growing older becomes a stark reality.

And what about the idea of dating at such an "advanced" age? After all, it's a little hard to pick up that stompin' stud at the latest Rave party when you can barely stay up past eleven o'clock at night anymore. And how are you supposed to compete with those hunky college studs when your 8 a.m.-to-8 p.m. workday leaves you little time to work out at the gym, let alone the stamina to make it to "last call" at the local pub? Ben Gay, anyone?

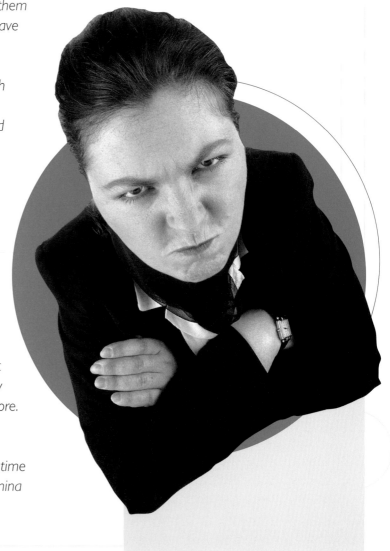

"HEY, WHO LET ALL THESE KIDS IN HERE?", OR: WELCOME TO YOUR PRE-MIDLIFE CRISIS

So, let's see. Everything still works, it just works slower. Everything's there, there's just too much of it. And what's gone, went fast! Hmm, sounds like somebody's having their midlife crisis a little early.

The human body, naturally, has physical limits that supersede those of caffeine, drugs, or alcohol, and, occasionally, gives its owner undeniable signs that it is tired of schlepping into the local faux-Irish pub or other nauseatingly decorated theme bar six nights out of seven a week.

Such signs include a queasy feeling when approaching one's cologne shelf in the medicine cabinet, accompanied by an irrational fear of bar stools or CD jukeboxes. Not to mention an intense desire to curl up on the living room couch and watch sober people prance around the boob tube in well-lit sit-coms where no one pukes in the restroom stall next to you or ends a sentence with ". . . it's not contagious as long as we use protection."

"Don't trust anyone over thirty who used to say 'Don't trust anyone over thirty'."
—Anonymous

It is as inevitable as the clothes you once laughed at coming back into style and the amount of hair in your brush each morning equaling that on your head. There comes a point in every modern single's life when their phase as a successful lounge lizard or barstool babe comes to an instant and irrefutable end. Usually it's when the beer, no matter how fresh or imported, tends to taste flat and the drink specials on the chalkboard by the door become harder

and harder to read, no matter how sober one is.

It is a moment defined by the simple observation made when you suddenly look around the crowded bar one evening and innocently ask yourself, "Hey, who let all these kids in here?"

It's not that you're too old, exactly. It's just that everyone else seems so *young*. They wear fashions that might as well be from another planet. Ask for drinks that sound more like porno movies than cocktails. Do things on the dance floor that you're sure are illegal in several states. Except for goatees and breasts, you can't tell which ones are boys or girls, especially when they kiss each other, which they do indiscriminately and without anything resembling rhyme or reason.

They play songs on the jukebox that defy explanation and speak a language so filled with modern allusions, inside jokes, and obnoxious slang that it barely approaches English except for an occasional "the" or four-letter word mixed in. Their retro cologne smells like hippie mothballs, and their cigarettes are foreign and thin.

They appear to clone themselves and multiply before your very eyes,

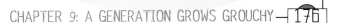

until you and the bartender appear to be the only sane members of society left on the planet. You commiserate over boring draft beers and take odds on which anorexic model wannabe will pass out first.

Despite the fact that you are a novelty due to your advanced age and excellent personal hygiene, the members of the opposite sex who occasionally hit on you are so boring and inane that you find it impossible to muster any attraction to them whatsoever.

And so, eventually, like the once proud king of the jungle put out to pasture with his gray mane and smacking gums, you will hand over your old watering hole to the glitter and the neon, the raves and the hip-hop, the clove cigarettes and the trendy drinks.

Like they say at last call, "You don't have to go home, but you can't stay here."

TOP-5 SIGNS YOU'RE TOO POOPED TO POP

5 Instead of your driver's license, the bouncer asks to see your AARP card.

4 Kids keep asking you if you've got any hits of Viagra on you.

3 Young girls keep telling you they haven't seen your daughter around here lately.

2 People keep asking you if this disco was anything like Studio 54.

1 That hottie you thought was flirting with you just wants your autograph, Mr. Cronkite.

DARTH DILEMMA: VADER VS. MAUL

They used to be called "May/December" romances, but with global warming, huge holes missing out of the ozone layer, and natural disasters no longer discriminating between normally recognized times of the year, are so-called seasons really even relevant anymore? Movies are a much more constant American standby, and while we may no longer be able to rely on the solstice, the moon, or the stars, we can always rely on *Star Wars*.

And so the question becomes, when you and your "mature" frame of reference favors Darth Vader and all of his implied doom, and your flashy new boy-toy would much rather watch Darth Maul, who picks up the tab for dinner?

Everything was going so well. Despite your age difference, he was funny, cute, had a good job, and never said a word about your cellulite. His stamina was amazing, even if a little unimaginative, and he always understood when you needed your space the next morning.

Fresh out of college, he was full of ideas and notions, goals and dreams, and his enthusiasm had leant new life to your own long-buried emotions. You often spent whole nights just talking, about anything and nothing at all, until the wine ran out and the sun came up, and you drifted off to sleep like two spoons nestled together in the silverware drawer.

Of course, your friends never missed an opportunity to point out your age difference, despite, or maybe because of, your obvious happiness. They were all quite certain nothing would come of your "illicit" romance, and wrote it off to pre-mid-life-pre-pre-menopausal jitters, despite your admonitions that this was the "real thing—finally."

Your mother, of course, had quit speaking to you ever since that little incident when you brought him over for the inevitable meet and greet. The one where he mistakenly referred to Jay Leno as the only *Tonight Show* host. Your father, a big Jack Paar fan, skipped dessert for the first time in sixty-four years.

Still, the two of you were content to stand, hand in hand, alone against the slings and arrows of the harsh, cruel world as you mentally calculated the age at which you would officially stop celebrating birthdays in order for him to catch up properly.

Everything was going smoothly, that is, until your usual Wednesday evening trip to the video store turned into a galactic explosion to rival that of the Death Star.

You'd seen all his artsy, angsty flicks and he'd seen all your tearjerkers, so to compromise you meandered into the science fiction aisle. Simultaneously, you each reach for *Star Wars.* Yours the original, his the prequel.

"Come on," you whine perkily, batting your eyelashes, a trick that usually still worked. "You're joking, right? If you think I'm sitting through that self-indulgent schlock again, you're crazy. I can't stand how flat the characters are and that little kid drives me crazy. And don't even get me started on that stupid Jar Jar Binks fool."

"That kid," he squeaks, reminding you of just how much closer he is to puberty than to posterity, "is the future Darth Vader! And he's the best child actor to come along since that kid from *Home Alone.*"

"Darth Vader?" you quip. "That little towheaded tyke's not fit to hold Vader's voice box. James Earl Jones always was, and always will be, Darth Vader. Everybody knows that."

"Vader sucks," he says passionately, the thin attempt at a goatee quivering along with his boyish chin, something you wish you would have noticed before. "Darth Maul would kick his tired old ass before you could say 'Jedi Knight.'"

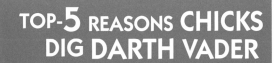

TOP-5 REASONS CHICKS DIG DARTH VADER

5 He can fondle them from across the room.

4 Who can resist a man in a cape?

3 Heavy breathing + big black mask = Va Va Voom!

2 The dark side always has more fun.

1 Three words: big light saber.

"You mean that sorry excuse for commercial merchandising that was still available for purchase at every Taco Bell and McDonald's eight months after the movie came out?" you accuse, watching the apples in his young cheeks turn into blazing coals.

"What do you know?" he spits, hitting below the belt. "Your tired, old eyes couldn't tell the difference between Darth Maul and Queen Amidala anyway."

"Old?" you shout, beyond Embarrassment-ville and wandering straight into Tantrum City. "I'll show you old."

With that, you march straight up to the video counter and request that your boy toy's name be stricken from your rental privileges forever. Whining next to you, he whimpers that he didn't mean it.

You nod at the video clerk nonetheless. She hits "delete" on her keyboard as you watch your ex-boyfriend, emphasis on "boy," fumble through his wallet for a major credit card to start his own account.

"But I don't have one," he whines to the clerk. "All I have is my 'Phantom Menace Fan Club' card."

As you leave the store with the clerk's laughter still ringing in your ears, you remember wistfully your boy toy's excellent stamina.

He'll need all of it for the walk home . . . alone.

DRIVE-THRU LONELY

For a simple way to tell if you are at the bottom or the top rung of your generational dating ladder, consider the following scenario, and then rate it on a scale of one to ten. One being "highly unlikely" and ten being "happened to me just yesterday":

It's payday and your boss, who's been promising to catch up with the millennium and actually look into that new-fangled concept known as "direct deposit," still hasn't quite gotten around to it. A thunderstorm worthy of a *Weather Channel Live Report* begins precisely at noon, and people who were otherwise just sitting at home and enjoying their day off suddenly jumped up and said, "I think I'll just run out to the bank for a sec!"

Standing in a line worthy of last summer's biggest blockbuster movie, you fill out your deposit slip on the back of your wallet and hope you didn't leave your headlights on. Meanwhile, a college kid behind you in mirrored shades and a weak goatee wrings out his Foo Fighters T-shirt on your $140 loafers as you try not to notice the pot scent wafting off of his three-day-old jean shorts and Birkenstocks.

You finish your deposit slip and ignore the kid, trying to concentrate instead on Ariel, the twenty-

something teller you've been lusting after for months now. Or at least ever since she let you cash a check that day the ATM was broken and she didn't even charge you for the teller visit, despite the fact that at thirty you're still on the budget checking account plan.

"She wants me," you thought, even though she's waited on you eighteen times since then without so much as even a flicker of recognition. Over the counter you can just see the silver belly-button ring blazing dully through the sheer white blouse. You wonder why the bank allows her to wear it, since you can see her black bra clearly as well.

She's talking patiently to a granny about her savings account and you quickly scan the seven customers in front of you, mentally doling them out to the other three tellers and quietly calculating the odds that you might just be lucky enough to have Ariel wait on you once again.

When you do, in one of those fateful moments that seem to happen so rarely now that you've quit taking Ecstasy, you wonder why she keeps looking over your slightly

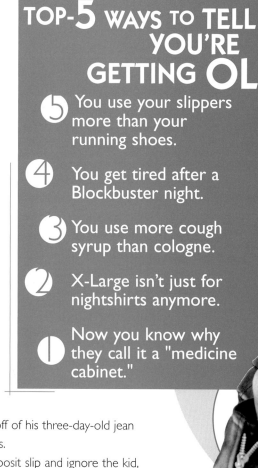

TOP-**5** WAYS TO TELL YOU'RE GETTING **OLD**

5 You use your slippers more than your running shoes.

4 You get tired after a Blockbuster night.

3 You use more cough syrup than cologne.

2 X-Large isn't just for nightshirts anymore.

1 Now you know why they call it a "medicine cabinet."

balding head. Ignoring the buxom bank teller's roving eyes, you make feeble money jokes and finger-comb your thinning hair as you tell her you've forgotten your account number . . . again. You haven't, of course, but there's just something about watching her purple-painted lips forming all of those non-sequential numbers that forces you to lie.

> "Gray hair is a sign of age, not wisdom."
>
> —Greek Proverb

Then you remember just exactly who was behind you: the pothead in the Birkenstocks. Her gaze shifts from just over your head to the left of you, as he slouches up to the only guy teller in the building and asks him for $180 back from his $200 paycheck from his part-time job at the local Kinko's. The guy reminds the kid that he signed up for the automatic $25 savings withdrawal, way back when. You smile when he says it, then watch Ariel's fleshy middle jiggle provocatively through her see-through shirt as she gets involved, leaving you high and dry while she sorts it out across the teller counter, her budding breasts heaving with every flirtatious giggle as the frat boy twists his limp goatee.

"Excuse me," you interject forcefully, remembering suddenly that you are, after all, an adult now and don't have to put up with this kind of thing anymore, "I'd like to speak with the manager, please."

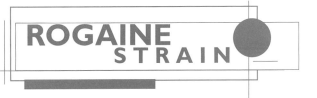

It's Saturday night and that cute girl from the gym finally let you ask her out. You spent all day trying to think about *not* thinking about your big date, jogging in the morning, shaving in the afternoon, until finally it was six o'clock and time for you to officially begin thinking about picking her up.

You've cleaned up your car and even bought one

of those pine tree air fresheners to try and get rid of the ever-present stench of those Wendy's to-go bags that had littered the passenger side floor until that very morning.

You find a jazz station on the radio and try not to get too scared when the current song stretches out for miles and you wonder if you've driven into a dating time warp. But she seems like the jazzy type to you, with her cute little bob haircut and mauve fingernail polish, and so you listen carefully as the DJ informs you that a group known as the Reefertons had just performed the last song. You remember the title, "Wafer Thin," hoping to impress her with your hep-cat knowledge during a late-night aperitif.

Wondering why a twelve-minute saxophone riff accompanied by acoustic guitar and bongos even needs a title in the first place, you realize that you've arrived in the direct vicinity of her street . . . completely empty-handed. No flowers. No candy. Not even a politically correct bag of recycled bird feed or a donation to UNICEF in her name.

Spotting a convenience store that's seen better days two streets past hers, you zip in for something to hand her when she opens the door. A gang of junior high hooligans leans against the cinder block wall under a sign that says, "Only two students at a time!" They snicker as you walk past, confirming your fear that you do indeed look like a dork after all in your pleated khakis and banded collar Hilfiger dress shirt.

But the slacks feel looser than ever and your new loafers make you an inch taller and besides, you'll never have another zit, wet dream, or afternoon detention in your life, so you puff up your chest as you walk by them and sneer your grown-up sneer.

Inside the store, air conditioning smacks you in the face and you find a seven dollar bottle of white zinfandel, since you don't yet know if she prefers white or red. And, even though any wine that starts with "z" is totally cheesy and she'll probably hate it, you'll still get brownie points for the effort. Besides, now she'll have something in the back of her fridge to serve that old college friend of hers that shows up unannounced one day, the one she never really liked anyway.

Standing in line between a woman who's never gotten a money order before but keeps telling everyone who'll listen that she needs it to pay the light bill and a construction worker eyeing the dirty magazines under the cigarettes with admiring grunts, you notice a slightly balding yuppie in the security camera behind you.

Smirking to yourself, you regard the butterflies on the sweaty wine label in your hand and thank God that isn't you. But, wait a second. Another quick glance confirms that the woman in front of the chrome dome geek is handing over the electric bill money and the mountain man covered in concrete dust behind Kojak is playing pocket pool—

TOP-5 POLITE WAYS TO GET YOUR MAN TO USE ROGAINE

5 "You know, I wouldn't have to wear sunglasses so much if that glare off the top of your head wasn't so blinding."

4 "I can't tell who you remind me of more, Ron Howard or his brother."

3 "Does your bald spot ever get cold?"

2 "Don't you think you're a little old for a baseball cap collection?"

1 "Dang, I forgot my compact. Can I use your head again?"

so that means … it *is* you!

You put the wine back in the beer cooler and exit the store immediately. At a store down the street, you buy yourself a box of Ring Dings and a Diet Mountain Dew, stopping at the pay phone out front to call the jazzy girl and complain of stomach cramps from too many crunches at the gym that morning. On the way home you wonder, "Now, is that nifty new sit-com on Friday night or Saturday?"

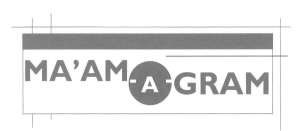

MA'AM-A-GRAM

It was bound to happen, no matter how long you may have avoided it or tried to deny it. Your young, hip clothes. The "new artists" stacked carefully in your CD collection, despite the fact that the names, such as "Korn" and "Screamin' Cheetah Wheelies," actually scare you. Even that little butterfly or snake tattoo hidden so cleverly on the back of your ever-widening ankle couldn't delay the inevitable.

None of that matters when the "kid" you were subtly, but not so subtly, flirting with in the line at the local grocery store or coffee shop approaches you cockily and says, "Excuse me, ma'am. I couldn't help but notice you winking at me for the last half hour, and I just wanted to ask, is there something in your eye?"

HILDA'S STORY

Hilda knew that the clock was ticking on the stopwatch so carefully hidden in her looks department. She'd noticed the word "gravity" slipping into her vocabulary every so often lately, as in, "I didn't used to need a bra with so much support—until gravity kicked in, that is."

Hilda was tired of watching seventeen-year-olds guzzle milkshakes and pies while their concave stomachs glared through between their flare jeans and little pink tube tops, even as her lunch salad pressed uncomfortably against the ever-tightening waistband of her size 12 slacks. She was tired of doing Tae-Bo every night after work and before her bland Lean Cuisine dinner.

Especially when three straight months of it had failed to eliminate the ever-present layer of cellulite covering the backs of her thighs, which she now only showed to intimate relatives and her family doctor.

She'd stopped buying fashion magazines long ago, but still felt guilty that she didn't look like a cover girl. She felt old long beyond her years, and couldn't understand why. It wasn't as if she wanted to attract a younger man, exactly. After all, they seemed exceedingly boring and preoccupied with music and fashion. But she couldn't stand to not even be in the running, either.

Her current boyfriend, Clyde, a thirty-two-year-old accountant with good teeth and bad skin, took it all in stride. He'd long since grown accustomed to walking beside her, not behind her, so that she wouldn't have to warn him against looking at, as she called it, her "fat ass." He was used to being interrupted in the middle of a completely non-sexual conversation with an

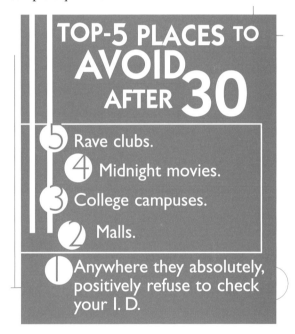

urgent, "You see that girl's boobs over there. They're fake."

He didn't even mind the "sex with the lights off," the "sex under the covers," or even the "don't touch my stomach, thighs, or butt during sex" rule.

But despite his good job and even better nature, Hilda secretly wished that, just once, Clyde would say, "But Hilda, you're not fat. You're not old. You're a beautiful, vibrant, exciting thirty-one-year old who makes my heart skip a beat each time you walk in the room."

Was that so hard? Clyde could crunch numbers all day long, find loopholes in software that saved his boss thousands of dollars, but he couldn't reassure a perfectly attractive female that she still had what it took to light his own fiscal fire?

"Few women admit their age. Few men act theirs."

—Random bumper sticker

Still, she guessed some of Clyde's current quietness was partly her fault. Long ago he had learned not to utter such platitudes as, "You look fine." Or, "Your butt looks exactly the same to me." Or, "You're right, black is slimming."

Her constant quip to such remarks was always a short, clipped, "Don't patronize me, Clyde." She guessed that he'd finally just grown tired of hearing it and so now simply said nothing.

So was it her fault that they broke up last week after stopping at the liquor store on the way home for some Kahlua to mix after dinner drinks with? After all, it had been another "pleasant" evening spent listening to Clyde talk about his job and then hearing his lame excuse why he'd left his wallet in his desk at work again.

She noticed he hadn't left his wallet anywhere but in his pocket when he bought that new laptop last week, or the $300 thermostat for the industrial size fridge in his immaculate garage where he brewed his own beer and needed "just the right temperature" for the new coffee porter he was experimenting with.

Still, Hilda was a modern woman and knew that there was nothing fair about being the "fairer" sex. So, of course, she bought dinner and caught all of Clyde's yawns, his inevitable sign that he was tired from yet another long week at work (like she wasn't?) and didn't have the energy to stop off at that little piano bar she liked so much. Was it too much to ask for one more nightcap before going back to her place where he'd fall asleep on the couch in front of the Sci-Fi channel?

As a compromise, he'd agreed to stop by the liquor store. Finding a ball game on the radio, he not only didn't help her out of the car, but settled in the passenger seat instead while she went inside alone.

Fuming, Hilda perused the endless aisles of brandy and specialty drinks at her leisure. Lingering over the funky margarita glasses and aged cheeses, she finally settled on a bottle of Kahlua and brought it up to the cashier.

A college kid with a buzz cut and peach fuzz rang up her purchase. She watched his long, pale fingers linger over the large, brown bottle as he scanned it into the register. Reaching for her credit card, she was surprised when he cleared his throat and in an unflinching voice asked, "Can I see some I.D.?"

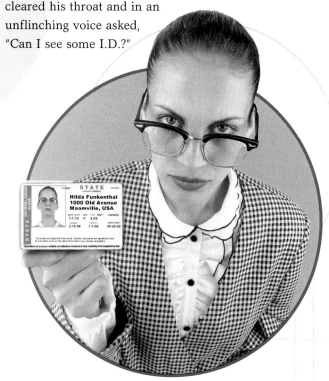

Looking into his jellybean green eyes, she blushed and said, "Excuse me?"

"Your driver's license," he said gently in a soft voice framed by straight, white teeth not more than five years out of braces. "Or any I.D. that says you're over twenty-one."

Looking quickly over her shoulder to make sure he wasn't addressing the teenybopper standing in line behind her, she fumbled quickly

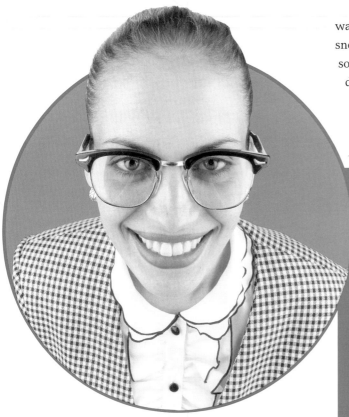

watery knees to her Toyota Camry to find Clyde snoring in his Dockers and Oxford shirt, she not so accidentally bumped the horn sliding into the driver's seat.

"What the—" he snorted, the drool on his chin glistening in the harsh, sodium glare of the liquor store parking lights.

TOP-5 WAYS TO MAKE A 30-SOMETHING FEMALE SMILE

5 "You know, the student discount is cheaper than the twilight show."

4 "Actually, the 'young miss' section is over there."

3 "Hi. I'm here to take your younger sister on a date."

2 "Is this your first time voting?"

1 "May I see your I.D., young lady?"

for her driver's license, suddenly eager to please this handsome stranger with the silver tongue.

"Wow," he said admiringly, and she hung her head in shame, assuming he had quickly found the early '70s birth date. Instead, he pleasured her again with the tender line, "I see a lot of driver's licenses in my line of work, and usually people take really crappy pictures. But yours looks like the cover of one of those girlie magazines."

Snapping her head up, she saw him blushing, quickly trying to find the right word. "That's," he sputtered, "not what I meant. I meant fashion magazines. You know, 'girls' magazines."

Back in her good graces, she gratefully accepted her I.D. back from the boy wonder and paid for her liqueur. Their fingers touched as he handed her the crinkly brown bag, and she felt more excitement in that one tiny moment than she had in years.

They shared a glance that could only be called "smoldering," something she thought had been put out in her years ago, and when she returned on

"Clyde," she said matter-of-factly on the short drive back to her place. "Thank you for putting up with me for the last four months, but, I think it's best when we get to my apartment if you don't come up. Ever again."

Clyde grunted, still sleepy, and kissed her gently on the cheek in the parking lot. Upstairs, she poured herself a Kahlua on the rocks and quietly contemplated all the wonderful excuses she could use to visit her neighborhood liquor store that week.

MAKING A
SPECTACLE

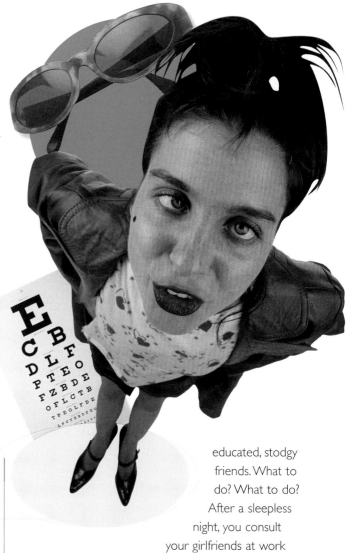

The e-mail sits there quietly, indiscriminate among the daily spam and "joke-a-day" lists that pile up by the time you finally drag yourself home from work.

"Hi, gorgeous," it reads, bringing an instant blush to your face. "I saw your picture in the company newsletter. (Don't try and guess, I got it from a friend.) Those cat woman glasses you had on are SO hip. Care to meet me for a drink tomorrow night after work? How about Mulligan's on Fifth and Central? I'll be your Superman, only dressed like Clark Kent. Signed, The Man of Steel."

Fanning yourself with your *Ally McBeal* mousepad, you read, then re-read, the message over and over again. The e-mail's sender is unfamiliar to you, the cadence, humor and grammar unlike any of your well-educated, stodgy friends. What to do? What to do? After a sleepless night, you consult your girlfriends at work over salads and diet colas in the break room.

"Go," they shout in unison, passing around your copy of the semi-erotic e-mail. "What have you got to lose? You haven't had a date in months!"

Sylvie, the redhead, volunteers to follow you into Mulligan's and scope out the situation until you give her a "thumbs up" or a "thumbs down," at which point she will either leave immediately and call you in the morning or pull the conveniently located fire alarm.

With nothing to lose, you while away the long, lonely hours at work before the whistle finally blows and you race into the ladies' room for a little primping before the short drive to Mulligan's.

A lemon daiquiri does little to soothe the butterflies in your stomach as Sylvie scouts the

TOP-5 SIGNS YOU MIGHT NEED GLASSES

5 You keep asking, "Who's this Janet Reno babe?"

4 You keep a magnifying glass next to your big screen TV.

3 You squint more than you blink.

2 You refer to your front row seats at the opera as "the nosebleed section."

1 Binoculars are a fashion accessory.

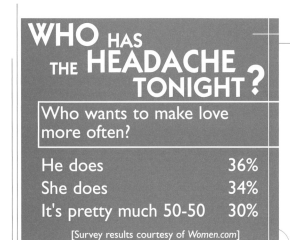

WHO HAS THE HEADACHE TONIGHT?

Who wants to make love more often?

He does	36%
She does	34%
It's pretty much 50-50	30%

[Survey results courtesy of *Women.com*]

crowd for that hunky Clark Kent. You munch beer nuts and watch CNN at the bar for an hour, slowly willing your heart not to break as Sylvie consoles you on her way out the door.

"Sorry, kid," she says earnestly. "But I've got kick boxing at seven and the instructor looks just like the guy who invented Tae-Bo. You wanna come with? It might get your mind off of being stood up by some creepy hacker."

"No," you tell her, signaling the bartender for your bill. "I'm just going to head home and cancel my e-mail account." She laughs as you watch her red hair bound out the swinging doors.

Moments later, a suave presence creeps up behind you amidst the rustle of his tweed jacket and the scent of his classy cologne and says in a voice as deep as the cold Atlantic, "I promise you, in bed I'm not faster than a speeding bullet."

Despite the cheesy comment, you're so relieved not to be stood up that you turn to face your secret admirer. His smile, once so prominent beneath his thick, horn-rimmed glasses, fades instantly.

"Hey," he pouts. "Where are those sexy glasses of yours I saw in the company newsletter?"

"Sexy?" you laugh. "I got rid of those nerdy things weeks ago. Don't you like my new contacts?"

You might just as well have asked if he enjoyed a good case of herpes!

"Contacts?" he practically shouts, waving away the bartender's request to take his drink order. "What decade

are you living in? Smell the coffee, honey. Look around you. Glasses are where it's definitely at. Check mine out—$200 and not a thing wrong with my eyes. Perfect 20/20 vision. But does the whole Clark Kent vibe fly? You betcha!" You listen as his voice trails off the more he loses interest.

Watching his khaki Dockers amble amiably over to a table of four-eyed females, you take a cue from his diatribe and glance around the crowded bar. Spectacles, glasses, shades, and even an eyepiece or two dot three out of four happy faces. Many squint through the heavy lenses just to see their neighbor or nearby drinking buddy, and you are quite positive that of the bespectacled majority, half again probably possess eagle eyes as good or better than your mystery man's.

If you were only still in high school, your years of therapy bills to battle eyeball insecurity and glasses-a-phobia could have been spent on a different pair of frames for each night of the week!

Who knew? Half expecting to be called a "nerd" yet again, only this time for the *opposite* reason, you dash from the bar and head for the nearest all night, one-hour Lenscrafters.

Maybe they'll have a two-for-one sale!

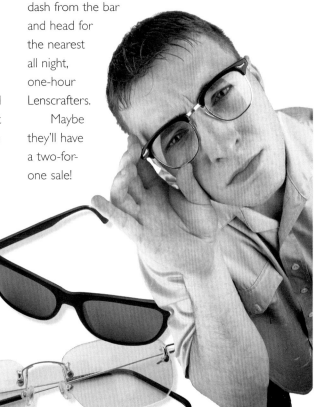

ALLY McBACKLASH

Blame it on *Ally McBeal*. Blame it on Courteney Cox. Blame it on *Will & Grace*. But no matter who you blame it on, the fact is that a certain segment of America is getting thinner, and not in a good way. We're talking skeletal, walking dead, one-foot-in-the-grave skinny. And it's not just those emaciated chicks in the cheesy Anorexia Nervosa after-school specials over on the Lifetime channel, either.

In another desperate attempt to stave off old age at any cost, many aging youngsters who wake up one morning to find themselves teetering on the brink of thirty (and beyond) choose to starve themselves in order to return to that formerly youthful thinness they see in past yearbook, graduation, and passport photos.

Let's face it, who else but gainfully employed twenty-somethings could afford all that Slim Fast anyway? Girls who spend their day glued to a computer monitor from a locked-in seated position find themselves burning calories at a much slower rate than they did cheerleading, jogging, and flirting back in school. But it's not just the ladies who are starving themselves in order to look "young again." Guys are doing it too. A few love handles is all it takes to push a formerly Jockey Joe into a Bulimic Bob these days!

Whether this is yet another case of "Ally McBacklash" or not, the trend is real and in no danger of vanishing anytime soon. In fact, many stubborn singles find themselves faced with a never ending sea of famished finds from which to choose their partners and mates. Which brings up the interesting question: Ladies, can you really date a guy who weighs less than you? As in, fifty *pounds* less than you?

TOP-5 TABLOID HEADLINES YOU'LL PROBABLY NEVER SEE

5. AUTOPSY RESULTS: ELVIS REALLY IS DEAD

4. EXPERT REVEALS TWO-HEADED ALIEN BABY REALLY JUST CLEVERLY RE-TOUCHED PHOTO!

3. STUDY SHOWS AMERICANS NOT QUITE AS STUPID AS WE THOUGHT!

2. TRY THE NEW MARLON BRANDO DIET!

1. OPRAH BROKE!

ANOREXIA
SPLURGOSA

It is your first real date and, for something original, you decided to offer to cook him dinner, at his place. Taken aback, he had agreed readily, impressed with your unbridled altruism and already salivating at the prospect of a home-cooked meal.

Guiltily, you chose not to reveal your true intentions, not the least of which was to feed this emaciated soul who'd bumped into you every day for a week in the coffee shop downstairs from your workplace and who looked as skinny as a vanilla bean and as pale as vanilla ice cream. Secondly, you wanted to check his medicine cabinets to see if his appalling thinness was a medical condition. Thirdly, of course, he seemed like the starving artist type and you were tired of taking guys out to dinner only to get stuck with the bill. At least this way you could save yourself a few bucks.

So, full of questions and bulging shopping bags, you show up at his inevitably artsy loft in a seedy section of town just in time to see him slipping into his silk shirt and leather pants through the window panel in the front door. Not turned on in the least, you realize he is even thinner than you had originally thought. That leather coat of his had puffed him out considerably. Here, half-naked in the dim light of a single bathroom bulb, his ribs were more prominent than one of those sick

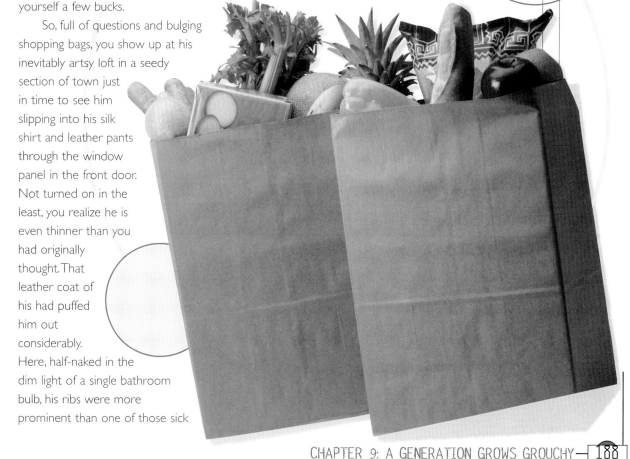

greyhounds you saw on the news every so often. His stomach looks about ready to greet his back it is so concave, and you find yourself wondering how he gets out of bed in the morning.

Answering the door, he gentlemanly helps you with the bags, or, at least, the light ones anyway. Watching you slice and dice, wash and peel, he pours you a glass of wine and slips in a decidedly funky CD to match his art deco-meets-drab apartment.

Over wine and cheese, which he barely touches, you ask him about himself. (Always a good icebreaker, you've learned.) In between cringing at his skinny fingers and thin lips, you decipher that he's a waiter at a restaurant up the street from your shared coffeehouse, but that his real passion is modeling.

"That explains it," you let slip, your tongue obviously loosened by wine and—disgust.

"Explains what?" he asks defensively, obviously realizing that you outweigh him by a good thirty pounds.

"Why you're so thin," you say, wanting everything out on the table, before you go through the work of preparing the meal, just in case he decides to kick you out early and save you the trouble.

"Well, yeah," he says proudly, sipping at his wine despite the fact that its level is the same as it was when he began drinking it. You are convinced he is spitting it back when you're not looking, the way you've heard anorexics will chew on egg whites before spitting them out, to get the protein but none of the calories. "That's what the agencies want. Thin is in. Plus, I'm not getting any younger, you know."

"Can I ask you?" you venture, since you're the one holding the knife, "Which agencies? I mean, are you working?"

"Actually," he blushes. "I'm sort of a struggling model. I've taken some head shots, talked to some people, but as of yet, I haven't done any real modeling."

"Listen," you say, finishing off your wine and pouring more for the both of you. "Nothing personal, but maybe you're talking to the wrong agencies. Because, unless you are into the female impersonation bit, you're too darn thin."

"Really?" he says in a cutish, puppy dog way. Make that, starving puppy dog way. "But everyone's told me thin is in."

"Yeah," you snort, chomping on a carrot. "If you want to look like death warmed over. As in 'Here's what can happen when you don't wear a condom.'

"Listen," you go on, sliding the cheese and cracker plate back in his direction ever-so-discreetly. "I like you. You're sweet. But there's no way we're ever going to bed unless you gain some weight."

He snorts into his wineglass, surprised at your honesty. "Really?" he flirts. "And why not, if you don't mind telling me?"

"Because," you admit. "I made a promise to myself never to sleep with anybody who weighs less than I do. And, by the looks of it, you've got about fifteen pounds to gain if you ever want to get anywhere past the first course."

"So," he considers. "It's either you in the sack or my modeling career—"

"Not really," you interrupt. "It works the same way. Unless you're modeling hospital gowns, no girl is going to buy what you're selling without a little meat on your bones. Trust me. I'm a sucker for a little beefcake, and I'm pretty sure I'm not alone.

"You stick with me," you conclude, knife in hand. "And I'll not only get you into bed, but through a few more modeling agencies' front doors as well."

"Deal," he says, and, looking down, you realize he's finished the cheese already! And, of course, you're flattered that he devours his meal and half of yours, before scarfing down the quart of ice cream you brought for dessert.

Until, you realize, he's probably doing it all for his career!

"Oh, well," you think as he undoes a button on his ridiculous leather pants to make room for his "bloated" belly. "At least I've saved another male model from a life of starvation and rejection."

Besides, you realize selfishly, you still have at least another fourteen pounds to go before you have to decide whether you want to sleep with him or not.

SARCASM
SPILLS OVER

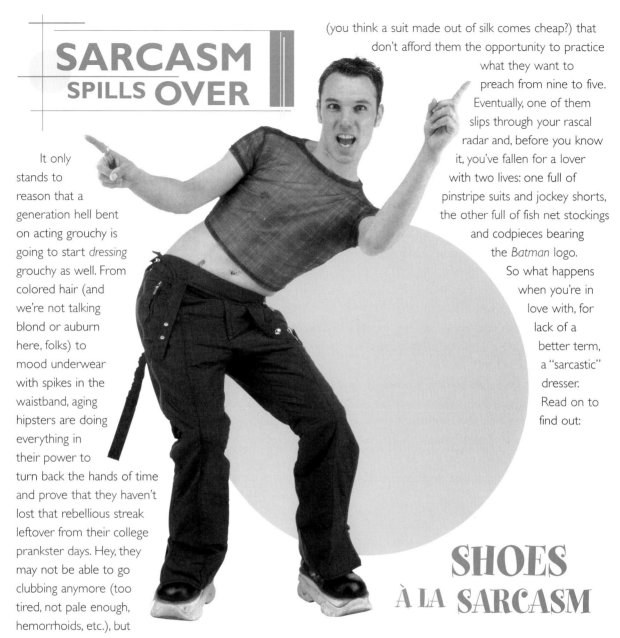

It only stands to reason that a generation hell bent on acting grouchy is going to start *dressing* grouchy as well. From colored hair (and we're not talking blond or auburn here, folks) to mood underwear with spikes in the waistband, aging hipsters are doing everything in their power to turn back the hands of time and prove that they haven't lost that rebellious streak leftover from their college prankster days. Hey, they may not be able to go clubbing anymore (too tired, not pale enough, hemorrhoids, etc.), but that doesn't stop them from wearing their Sid 'n Nancy shirts and pink and green plaid shorts to the mall come Saturday morning.

Fine. Dandy. Super. But what does all of this have to do with dating? Let's face it, as a generation grows grouchy, many of them remain single. (Just like you!) It's a simple equation, really: Bad Attitude + Bad Clothes = One Bad Case of Celibacy! Still, that doesn't mean that sarcastic dressers don't masquerade as normal looking, even attractive single and successful bachelors and bachelorettes. Many of them hold down awesome jobs

(you think a suit made out of silk comes cheap?) that don't afford them the opportunity to practice what they want to preach from nine to five. Eventually, one of them slips through your rascal radar and, before you know it, you've fallen for a lover with two lives: one full of pinstripe suits and jockey shorts, the other full of fish net stockings and codpieces bearing the *Batman* logo.

So what happens when you're in love with, for lack of a better term, a "sarcastic" dresser. Read on to find out:

SHOES
À LA SARCASM

Your current boyfriend is very cute, very clever, very smart, very sweet, very kind, very generous, very loving, very good in bed and, unfortunately, very sarcastic.

Everything he does is philosophical in some way or another. He's big into recycling, which is fine, except when done to extremes, which is how he does everything.

"No," he'll say, dragging you around town on one of his antiqueing missions on a Saturday morning, since he refuses to shop in any corporate owned store, which, according to him, is *any* store bearing a neon sign, security cameras, or indoor plumbing. "We can't stop at 7-11 and get coffee in a *Styrofoam* cup."

He says the word like it's a dirty one, and you're so caffeine starved, since he has to do everything at the crack of dawn, that you'd drink coffee out of a human skull if you had to. "We'll go to the natural food store and get you some coffee bean extract in a couple of hours."

He loves getting up on stage and ranting at local poetry readings, where you sit in the back, blushing and stooping below the scarred café table pretending to look for a fallen penny the entire time. Actually, however, he has a very respectable job managing one of the local video store chains, which he justifies (to himself, anyway) by never rewinding any of the videos that get turned in.

"There," he says gleefully after yet another shift. "That'll show 'the man.' Hmph."

Of all his sarcastic ways, however, his fashion statements speak the loudest. Pink Hi-Tops are somehow, to him anyway, symbolic. As are camouflage tank tops, satin boxers emblazoned with the *Superman* logo, baseball caps bearing only a question mark, plaid golf slacks with a white belt, old bowling shirts, stolen 7-11 and Wal-Mart aprons, and, of course, boxing trunks over bike pants.

Each eccentric outfit attests to, what he calls his "unique individuality and stereotypical outrage!" When you tell him he simply looks foolish, he counters with, what else, a sarcastic grin and a single word: "Exactly!"

You've put up with all of his "save the world" shenanigans for so long because, to be quite honest, you only see him on the weekends and once or twice a week, and, in short doses, he's quite delightful. When he's not being so sarcastic, that is.

But now you've been invited to the boss' annual summer barbecue and, in no uncertain terms, it has been suggested that all employees bring their significant

others. So you tell him, in said certain terms, that there is to be absolutely, positively *no* sarcasm displayed in his outer- or, for that matter, under-wear.

You insist on complete apparel approval and tell him that, should he fail you in this one and only instance, you will withhold sex for the rest of his natural life and burn every single sarcastic outfit in his closet without guilt, pity, or remorse.

He smiles, rather unsarcastically it appears to you, and agrees post haste. Which, naturally, makes you quite suspicious. Come the big night, he arrives wearing khaki Dockers, a white-collar shirt, and, stop the presses: a tweed blazer.

There is no Charlie Manson necktie, like the one he wore to meet your parents. No pink dye in his hair. No tuxedo or fake muscles T-shirt. No mood rings, fake moustaches, or hoop earrings bearing holy crosses. No Mr. T necklaces weighing down his neck or even the unmistakable scent of women's perfume.

Could he really be taking this seriously?

"Naw," you think, instructing him to drop his drawers in your well-lit foyer, as you are quite sure that he is wearing some type of exploding or otherwise embarrassing underwear. Or boxer shorts that, once in the presence of charcoal or barbecue sauce, instantly light up and say, "Corporate America Sucks!" or some other such subversive slogan that would no doubt offend your extremely corporate American boss.

Blushing, he complies, revealing his only too-staid *X-men* undies and nothing more.

"While my pants are around my ankles . . ." he quips as you gather up your purse and car keys.

"Maybe later," you promise. "If you're good."

"Oh," he grins, only

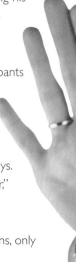

slightly sarcastically (you notice quite proudly), "I'm always good." Even his jokes are decidedly corny tonight. You smile, realizing he must actually like you after all.

In fact, your sarcastic boyfriend is decidedly subdued once at the party. He shakes your boss' hand firmly, but not too strongly. Does not flirt with any of the overly friendly gals from the secretary pool, and purposefully avoids coming too close to the kidney shaped swimming pool for fear of launching himself deep inside in spite of his good intentions.

He is charming, graceful, gentlemanly, and even listens to Harry from accounting's Vietnam War stories with a compassionate, if slightly glazed, look. You reward him with a heaping plate of baby back ribs and butter-drizzled corn on the cob, guiding him gratefully away from "Hanoi Harry," as he is known around the office, and steering him straight into two vacant lawn chairs.

Satisfied that the evening has been a success and that there will be nothing but glowing reviews of your "significant other" around the water cooler come Monday morning, you munch contentedly on smoked pork and try to ignore the twitters, gasps, silver dollar sized eye balls, and the hands raised to mouths directly across the lawn from you.

Wondering if your boyfriend had somehow managed to tear a seam in his pants or, possibly, unzip his fly, you regard him casually, noticing only a butter-smeared grin on his devilishly handsome face. His shirt is still buttoned, his jacket still tweed, his khakis still on, and nothing is unseemly about him except his insistence on crossing one leg, and then the other, rapidly, only to repeat himself over and over again.

"Sweetheart," you mouth around savory pig meat, "There are Porta-potties as far as the eye can see. If you need to use one, please just excuse yourself and go, for God's sake. Otherwise, quit fidgeting."

Wordlessly, you watch as he slows his leg

crossing machinations, but in no way, shape, or form quits them altogether. Excusing yourself for another ear of corn, supposedly, you stand up and cross the lawn to see what all of the businessmen and their wives are gawking at.

When you do, of course, you unceremoniously drop your Styrofoam plate on the boss' immaculate lawn and gasp at the single word, "SCREW" written in black, waterproof marker on the bottom of his left shoe, and the word "YOU!" written on the bottom of his right.

Snatching him up by the collar and dragging him to the car, you excuse yourself and apologize to every Tom, Dick, and Harriet from work along the way. Peeling out, you scold your now ex-boyfriend in every way imaginable, not buying for a minute his lame excuse. The one where he'd borrowed the shoes from his twin brother (whom you've never even heard about before) and had no idea the jerk had written nasty statements on their soles.

Dropping him off at his place, you peel out yet again and head for home. Later that night, however, once you've left yet another apologetic message on your boss' voice mail at work, you can't help but giggle over your beaux's subversive tactics.

And, even later that night, you have a dream in which your boyfriend becomes a successful entrepreneur, beginning with his own line of "sarcastic shoes." Waking up the next morning, you send him a sleepy e-mail before you chicken out. While sex is definitely out of the question, for now anyway, you wouldn't mind seeing him show up at your door one last time in that pair of boxer shorts you always thought were kind of cute.

The ones with the little happy, smiley faces . . . each one with a perfectly morbid contact wound gunshot directly in the center of its bloody forehead.

10

WORKPLACE WOOING
AND OTHER LAST RESORTS

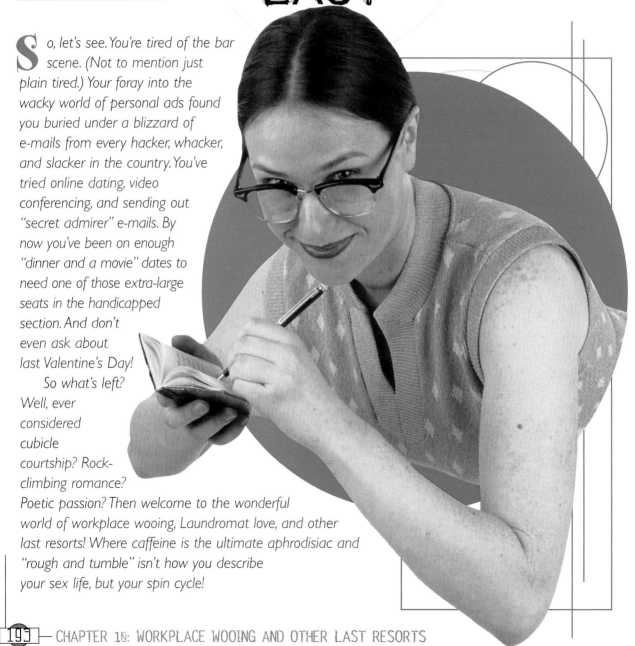

S o, let's see. You're tired of the bar scene. (Not to mention just plain tired.) Your foray into the wacky world of personal ads found you buried under a blizzard of e-mails from every hacker, whacker, and slacker in the country. You've tried online dating, video conferencing, and sending out "secret admirer" e-mails. By now you've been on enough "dinner and a movie" dates to need one of those extra-large seats in the handicapped section. And don't even ask about last Valentine's Day!

So what's left? Well, ever considered cubicle courtship? Rock-climbing romance? Poetic passion? Then welcome to the wonderful world of workplace wooing, Laundromat love, and other last resorts! Where caffeine is the ultimate aphrodisiac and "rough and tumble" isn't how you describe your sex life, but your spin cycle!

OFFICE ROMANCE: JUST THE FAX

There is an inevitable dry spell in between your clubbing phase and the desperation to go the personal ad route. This is, naturally, a period when you begin to seriously consider the workplace as a viable dating alternative. Usually this occurs only after you have sufficiently exhausted any and all other avenues of dating, including but not limited to: blind dates, friendly, well-intentioned set-ups proposed by in-laws, and church-organized prison visitations.

Accordingly, potential suitors to be found at the workplace are necessarily held to an entirely different set of standards than those found almost anywhere else. Fashion, of course, is thrown out the window since, you assume (and hope), that few people dress on the weekend the way they do at work. (Unless, that is, your occupation is a lingerie model.) Behavior is also afforded similar leeway, since you would hope that they do not behave at home the way they do at work—for example, photocopying their face or hands as a "fun" office gag.

The workplace romance is one of those "phases" most people go through on their way to better, truer love. It is something most people say they'll never do, even though most people end up doing so at one time or another. In many ways, as you grow older at least, it is in some ways … inevitable. Like noisy neighbors or lines at the Saturday night movies, workplace romance is just a modern fact of life that many singles grudgingly acquiesce to eventually.

Office romance, of course, is usually borne out of a hybrid sense of convenience and desperation, with just the slightest dash of laziness thrown in for good measure. There's an element of safety, as well. Unlike meeting a girl in a bar, let's say, a girl who might just be a front for a huge pharmaceutical conglomerate that specializes in slipping mickeys into unsuspecting guys' drinks and then expertly removing their kidneys before

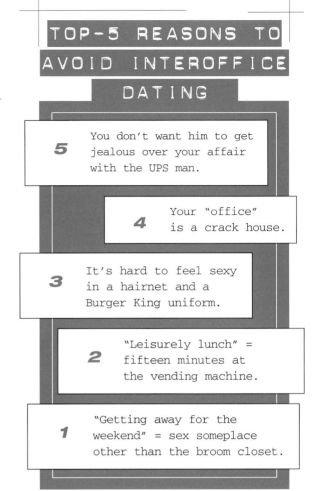

TOP-5 REASONS TO AVOID INTEROFFICE DATING

5 You don't want him to get jealous over your affair with the UPS man.

4 Your "office" is a crack house.

3 It's hard to feel sexy in a hairnet and a Burger King uniform.

2 "Leisurely lunch" = fifteen minutes at the vending machine.

1 "Getting away for the weekend" = sex someplace other than the broom closet.

they wake up the next morning, the co-worker in question has usually been observed for months or at least weeks in advance of actually going out with him or her.

You usually know whether or not said co-worker has an overabundance of tattoos or body odor, let's say. Other questions, naturally, are answered as well. Are the cops waiting by his Ford Taurus in the parking lot after work most days of the week? Is there an overabundance of flowers on her desk sent from Mafia bigwigs? Does he scratch himself incessantly? Does she keep a gun in her desk drawer?

These are all facts you would not have at your disposal in a blind date situation, for example. So there's that. There's also, depending on your work environment, a sense of similarity involved. If you can both work at the same place and actually survive, chances are a date will be no problem for either of you.

The date itself, of course, is another matter of convenience. Not only will the two of you likely choose someplace close to work, so that no one has to pick up or drop off anybody in case disaster strikes, but at least you'll always have something to talk about during those otherwise awkward pauses: work!

Of course, if things do go well and the two of you actually hit it off, the workplace romance is the best of both worlds. The two of you could conceivably spend twenty-four-hours a day together, indefinitely. There are the cute but spicy intra-office e-mails. Little sticky notes stuck on computer monitors with hearts and secret codes for dirty words. Sodas, teddy bears, or flowers left on desks while every lunch hour together is sixty minutes of bliss.

However, if something goes wrong, an eight-hour workday can soon feel like an eternity. When he turns into a selfish, cheap, egotistical jerk, which, for some reason, she couldn't see before they were out of the office, there is nothing much to do but avoid him and hope he has a short memory.

"Men always want to be a woman's first love. Women like to be a man's last romance."

– Oscar Wilde

When she catches him flirting with another girl around the office, there's not much for him to do but admit that he's a jerk and move on, or hide for the next seven and one-half hours.

It is at these times that the workplace becomes even more oppressive than ever, at least until the inevitable break-up period passes and the two former lovers can look forward to a long period of friendship based on shared experiences and cubicle lust.

Speaking of which, there is a danger element to workplace wooing that exists under a boss or manager who frowns on such things. In this case, short-term is obviously the way to go, as long-term romances, as detailed in the above paragraph, are often doomed from the outset. This is not a suggestion to make-out in the broom closet. However, seeing a co-worker on the sly while the rest of the office is blissfully unaware does have the exciting appeal of danger to it, and such feelings can often pass for passion in a pinch.

CUBICLE COURTSHIP: RAINBOW ROOM

Dating a co-worker is a little like buying milk at a convenience store. Sure, it's easy, but like the $4 you pay for a carton that's about the size of what they used to give you in second grade, the price can be high.

Consider the following cautionary tale:

A single guy, we'll call him "Dave," was growing

tired of the bar scene and too many well-intentioned, yet comical, set-ups by his so-called friends. There was a girl at work who was sort of cute. Although they weren't exactly the best of friends, he said "Hi" to her in the halls, and he once stood next to her in line at the company picnic, blathering on about baked beans and wondering if he'd put on deodorant that morning.

He liked the way her calves flexed on the way to the coffee machine every morning and that she didn't wear the corporate uniform of so many working girls: butterfly blouse, solid color skirt with anklets, and a pair of Nikes over her wheat-colored panty hose.

"In a great romance, each person plays a part the other really likes."

— Elizabeth Ashley

She was a little too fond of blazers with crests, but other than that, she was a far sight better than the dates he'd been having lately. So one day he decided to ask her out. He tried to do it Monday, but wondered that she might say "yes" just to be polite, thus allowing herself the rest of the week to think of an excuse why not to go after all.

He tried again on Tuesday, but wondered if she'd be hurt that he hadn't asked her on Monday. Then he decided to wait until Wednesday, figuring it might seem more casual that way, while still only giving her forty-eight hours to think of a polite way to stand him up.

But she was at a computer class on Wednesday and, he assumed, the next day as well, but when she waved to him in the parking lot after lunch on Thursday, he was too shocked and unprepared to even consider the script he'd written for himself.

Before he knew it, it was Friday and the thought of another boring weekend that would only culminate in the memories of bad movies and two dried out pizza boxes come Monday morning finally drove him to action. He bought her a diet soda from the break room, but when he went to drop it off, she wasn't there.

In the meantime, he stood just inside the "doorway" to her gray cubicle, admiring the rainbow

motif she had going on inside. There were rainbow posters touting inspirational sentiments like: "Success just wouldn't be the same without U!" A rainbow mug sat on a rainbow coaster while rainbow pencils sat in a cloud-shaped pencil holder. Rainbow stickers cluttered the bottom of each of her employee handbooks and memo folders, and when he'd waited fifteen minutes without her return, he scribbled a quick note on a rainbow pad and taped it to the soda, placing both on her rainbow mousepad to be sure she saw them. "Dear Hestia," it read, "I'll trade you a diet Coke for a date tonight? Yours truly, Dave, in accounting."

He felt relieved when he returned to his desk, thinking that he had the best of both worlds. He had asked her out without actually speaking, always a plus, and if she accepted, well, that was great. If not, hopefully

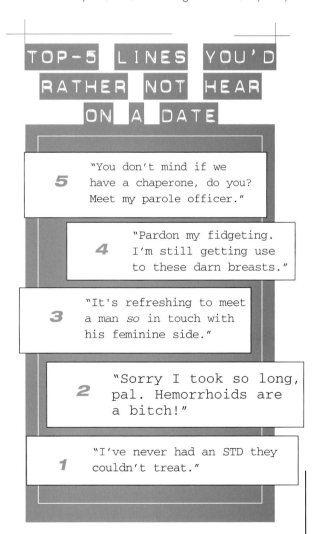

TOP-5 LINES YOU'D RATHER NOT HEAR ON A DATE

5 "You don't mind if we have a chaperone, do you? Meet my parole officer."

4 "Pardon my fidgeting. I'm still getting use to these darn breasts."

3 "It's refreshing to meet a man *so* in touch with his feminine side."

2 "Sorry I took so long, pal. Hemorrhoids are a bitch!"

1 "I've never had an STD they couldn't treat."

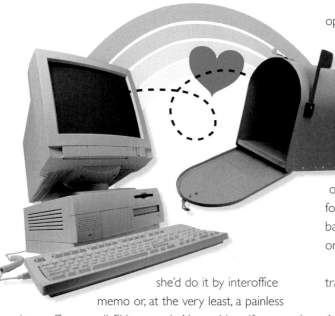

she'd do it by interoffice memo or, at the very least, a painless intra-office e-mail. Either way, he'd save himself an actual confrontation with a real, live human being.

But she surprised him by wandering into his cubicle several hours later, the rainbow sticky note blurred and running from the diet soda's condensation. "I was in a meeting," she smiled, "and all I could read of this note was 'Dave, in accounting.' Did you need something?"

"Just . . . j-just . . . you t-t-to accompany me on a date tonight?" he blurted, adrenaline taking over his bodily functions and shutting off the self-editing tool usually employed by his otherwise literate brain. Had he really said, "accompany?"

He was encouraged to see her blush, and even more so when she nodded and handed him back his soggy note.

There followed a brief flurry of e-mails confirming time and place, followed by a delightful evening spent in a noisy restaurant on opposite sides of a comfortable booth. There was the usual give and take, followed by a huge bitch session about work, always a nice icebreaker. The wait for a table in non-smoking must have been longer than they thought, for when he signed off on the bill his watch actually read 10:30! Why, it seemed like they'd only had minutes together.

And, after all, wasn't that the true sign of a good date? What had he been so worried about? Interoffice dating was, well, for lack of a better term, good.

He drove her to her apartment building, glad she lived on the third floor so that he didn't even have the

option of just "watching" her inside, but had to walk her up instead. She was flattered. They arrived at her door, where he saw a rainbow welcome mat outside her door as she fiddled with the keys. Expecting a quick, "good night," he was surprised to see her click on the hallway light and simply walk on in, obviously expecting him to follow.

He did so, but soon was overwhelmed. Rainbows in the kitchen, rainbows in the foyer, rainbows in the living room, rainbows in the bathroom. There were rainbows on the wall, rainbows on the floor tile, rainbows on the ceiling.

A fear clutched his throat. Had he suddenly been transported back to work?

Unfortunately, he hadn't—he'd crossed that line. And he'd crossed it with (insert that hokey *Twilight Zone* music here) "the girl whose apartment looked just like her cubicle."

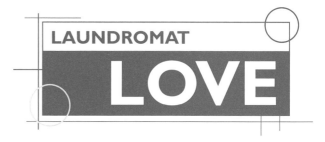

LAUNDROMAT LOVE

Of all the unspoken, great places to meet modern singles, the Laundromat is the dating version of that perfect, secret fishing hole you share with only your best friends. Unfortunately, all of their best friends and their best friends' friends and sisters, aunts, uncles, and cousins soon learn about it. Before long, your secret fishing hole looks like Venice Beach on a warm summer day and the only thing left to catch there is a good dose of noise pollution.

Once upon a time, Laundromats were like speakeasies or outlet stores, hidden finds where, when one showed up at the right place at the right time, one could find romance before the first spin cycle. However, like all good things in the information age, the rest of the world soon caught on.

Crafty Laundromat owners soon realized more was going on under their water-stained ceiling tiles than mere folding and fluffing. Despite the grumbling of some of their older customers, who actually came to the Laundromat to do *laundry,* renovations were soon underway. Gone was the mushroom and daisy wallpaper of the '60s. No more were the orange and industrial green plastic chairs from the '70s. The pork rinds and Slim Jims in the vending machine made way for Snackwell cookies and fat-free chips, and RC Cola eventually tipped its hat to Diet Coke.

Nowadays, many Laundromats even serve beer and wine, have air conditioning and track lighting, and actually cater to the singles crowds with cozy booths for two and smooth R&B pumped in over the Muzak. Names like "The Suds Shop" and "Brew and Bubbles" read more like singles bars than cleaning establishments, and doing one's laundry has become less of a chore and more of an opportunity.

After all, with all of that bright lighting, it's almost impossible to make the fluff-and-fold faux pas of hitting on a married woman. Why, her diamond ring would surely cause a glare in the glowing fluorescence. More important, the only time a married woman enters a Laundromat in the first place (unless, of course, she's looking for something decidedly more dirty than her husband's soiled underwear) is if her washer and dryer back home are broken.

In which case, of course, desperate to avoid being swarmed by the leering Laundromat lechers, she usually announces her presence with some bold declaration like, "Boy, I haven't been in a *Laundromat* since before I got *married* four years ago!"

Such a statement usually erects a force field of indiscriminate proportions around said married woman until she hefts her wicker laundry basket full of primly folded jockey shorts and baseball uniforms and then heads back out to her station wagon.

Laundromats are a lot like the waiting rooms of

pediatricians: There's lots to look at, pick up, and talk about, so that the kids don't get too scared of the needles, tongue depressors, and prescriptions waiting for them just on the other side of the door. Similarly, there are plenty of ways to strike up a conversation in a Laundromat.

Asking for quarters, of course, is probably the most obvious. First timers usually get shot down with a scalding glare and a turgid female (wedding ring-less) finger pointing to the sleek, black change machines dotting every three feet of the Laundromat's floor space. However, this is a mistake that's rarely made twice. Most guys (or gals) make sure to bring their crummiest, wiltiest, ripped-up-and-taped-back-together-poorly dollar bills to ensure that none of the change machines will ever take them.

Signs of receptiveness to this line are simply black

TOP-5 WORST LAUNDROMAT PICKUP LINES

5 "I was just admiring all of your dirty panties. Can I borrow a pair?"

4 "I just wrote you the sweetest love poem in the men's room. Care to read it with me?"

3 "I still have three minutes in final spin. You busy?"

2 "I'm looking for a new bleach. Who does your hair?"

1 "Can I borrow a quarter? I used all mine in the condom machine."

fabric softeners for the dryer.)

Subliminally, of course, detergent is the much better way to go than quarters. Money matters are never a great way to start a conversation, and if a guy can't even afford to do his own laundry, where are the happy but penniless couple supposed to have their first date? A few steps over at the vending machine? Detergent, however, just naturally leads to more maternal instincts.

"The most exciting attractions are between two opposites that never meet."

— Andy Warhol

"Oh," the uninitiated female might think, "he may have run out of detergent, but at least he's doing his laundry. Therefore, he's the responsible sort. How nice." Never mind the fact that his industrial size, warehouse tub of Tide is currently making his Honda Accord list to the left out in the brightly-lit parking lot just in case his amorous askings go unheard.

Regardless of the come on, however, once contact has been established, whether it be through quarters or bleach, hangers, or detergent, the next step is always so much easier at a Laundromat.

"How about a date?" he might ask across the cigarette stained folding table. "I have a thought," she might counter instead, carefully folding her bras behind the protective shelter of her laundry basket so as not to entice him any further. "Why don't we meet here next week at the same time. Then we can have dinner somewhere after our laundry's done and you won't have to pick me up."

Both parties win in this situation, of course. The guy has a date, and the girl has all week to find another

and white. A girl who's seeing someone or simply leery about meeting yet another Laundromat regular will always bring exact change. If she does have extra quarters, they're for the soda machine or a few games of Ms. Pac Man. Most single Laundromat goers, however, always have backup quarters just in case an unexpected hunk or hottie hits on them, in which case they're more than willing to give up the soda or, at the very least, the video games.

Desperate singles, of course, are as easy to spot as a bright orange Tide box. They're the ones with the Crown Royal bag bulging with enough quarters to supply a small bank or Brink's truck!

If asking for quarters fails, however, there is always detergent, or, in a pinch, bleach or possibly a coat hanger to request. (Rarely will a guy ask for one of those fluffy

Laundromat. Unless, of course, she sucks up the courage to actually return one week later and go through with it, in which case she has her own car to escape in if things go horribly at dinner. And, if things go really badly, she has at least a week's worth of clothing with her if she needs to skip town!

One-night stands are easier to achieve at a Laundromat as well, simply because a girl doesn't have to hide a "next morning" change of underwear in her oversize purse. She's got several pairs at her disposal, not to mention an entire wardrobe if it's a weeknight and there's work to go to the next morning.

The alcohol factor, or rather, the lack of it, is a problem, however. But half of the battle, the eye contact, the flirting, the one-liners, the come-ons, and the first impressions are already out of the way. The happy couple, their respective chores done for the evening, can always simply head for a nightcap on the way to his or her place.

Of course, like workplace or guy-from-the-apartment-next-door romances, breaking up with a Laundromat lover is always a potential problem. Laundromats, like corner bars, tend to inspire loyalty in their customers and switching over is a real pain in the butt. How far is it from home? What kinds of magazines do they have? Is the restroom clean? How often do they restock the gumball machine? These are all-important factors in the comfort level while washing clothes.

So, you must always be considering in the back of your mind, no matter how attractive the hunk or hottie in front of you: Are they worth the trouble of relocating if the relationship goes south?

If so, be liberal with your quarters, detergent, bleach, or eye contact. But if not, keep your quarters close to your vest and bury your head in last year's *People* magazine.

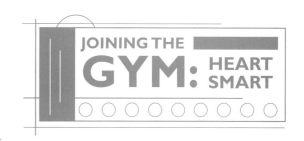

JOINING THE GYM: HEART SMART

Joining the local gym is yet another potentially pleasant, or possibly pungent, option for today's modern singles who are seeking a better-lit alternative to the usual dating scene than most dingy bars or cozy coffeehouses. For one thing, the dress code can be significantly more relaxed (and inexpensive) than most

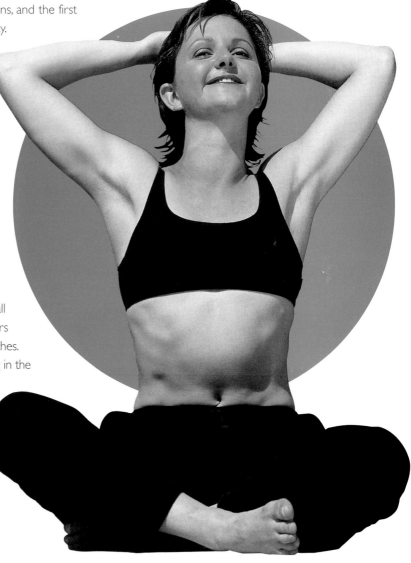

nightclubs or restaurants. In addition, there's nothing sexier than good, old-fashioned sweat. Especially when said sweat turns your lackluster 6 p.m. jazzercise session into a veritable wet T-shirt contest!

And where else can you stand behind a two-way mirror and watch your potential partner duking it out with an imaginary opponent while some cut-rate Tae-Bo instructor puts them through the motions as they jiggle and jive in nothing more than running shorts or a clingy leotard? Why, it might just be the socially acceptable version of drilling a peephole in the locker room wall.

"There is nothing better for the spirit or the body than a love affair. It elevates the thoughts and flattens the stomach."

– Barbara Howar

Furthermore, as opposed to many other dating activities that revolve around evening hours, the gym opens up an entirely new world for "daytime daters." Jogging around the indoor track on your lunch hour? Why not fall into step with that cute guy with the stopwatch? A quick comment on his running shoes, "Wow, are your feet *really* that big?" and he's likely to take a dive into the rubbery, faux-pebbles of the track's expensive, cushioned surface. When he gets up, however, there's all the more reason to stay by his side for the duration of his suddenly abbreviated run. The possibilities in such a case are endless.

If you can't wait for lunch to try out your fitness flirtations, however, there's always that "on-the-way-to-work" session where a few regular die-hards show up each morning. This provides an opportunity to set up an "after-work" date before you even get to the office, thus giving you all day to either look forward to said date, or think up an excuse why not to go: "Uh, yeah, Rico? Listen, I'd love to join you at that Air Supply concert tonight, but I think I pulled a hamstring when I was spotting you this morning." Another benefit of the "early bird" gym date is that, should

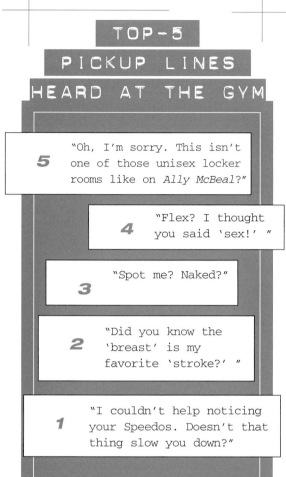

TOP-5
PICKUP LINES
HEARD AT THE GYM

5 "Oh, I'm sorry. This isn't one of those unisex locker rooms like on *Ally McBeal*?"

4 "Flex? I thought you said 'sex!' "

3 "Spot me? Naked?"

2 "Did you know the 'breast' is my favorite 'stroke?' "

1 "I couldn't help noticing your Speedos. Doesn't that thing slow you down?"

obvious, way to open up a line of conversation. One quick comment like, "Do you think you could spot me?" could lead to all kinds of opportunities, for men and women alike. Not only is this an instant partnership, but where else can you get a preview of a future partner's grunts and groans in broad daylight? Just be sure not to load on too much weight, however. Unless, that is, you want to spend your first date at the emergency room.

Other areas of the gym, naturally, are more prone to lend themselves to clever come-ons and pumped-up pick-up lines than others. The sauna is a natural, of course. Anything involving sweat, heat, towels, and a closed door is bound to stir up the hormones in even the most stubborn singles. If the sauna's too crowded, however, the lap pool is another natural. Speedos? "Breast"-strokes? Water? Goggles? Whistles? Need we say more?

Of course, when you're looking for love inside of a gym, timing is everything. (And we're not talking curl reps or cycling rotations, either.) Is that little hottie you've had your eye on for the past few weeks taking a break to head to the water fountain? Join her. Say something about her "form" on the Stairmaster and see if she's willing to put off another four floors of stepping to chat with you for a while.

Is that stud you've been drooling over all sweat session heading over to the treadmills? Is the one next to his

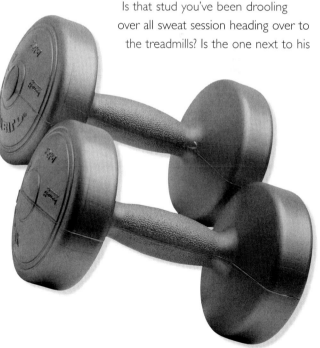

things progress smoothly and an eventual one-night stand is accomplished, you're sure not to have to make breakfast for your pectoral partner. After all, they'll more than likely be on the way to the gym before sun-up. If they do linger for some post-coital cookin', however, a quick Power Bar will more than likely do.

Of course, you have to be careful with such deltoid dates. After all, should anything go wrong and the two of you hard-bodies should actually break up, one or the other of you is going to have to change their workout schedule. Well, it's either that, or run the risk of getting a free weight dropped in your crotch the next time you're doing sit-ups.

Speaking of free weights, they are a quick, if

vacant? Who cares if you've already done six miles tonight, head on over. Fall into a rhythm and casually mention something about his snazzy running shoes. (Guys love it when you talk about their feet.)

Of course, no true gym rat can resist showing off his or her prowess on the equipment. So, even if you're a part-time aerobic instructor and know the exercise bikes in and out, from washers to warranty, go ahead and ask him to show you the "proper" way to ride one. Chances are, he'll be more than happy to help you. Especially when you take to it so fast thanks to his "expert" advice.

Guys, don't be afraid to use this tactic yourself. There's nothing sexier than a man strong enough to admit that he doesn't know how to set the caloric output gauge on his streamlined rowing machine. So ask away. Who knows, she may just "sail" right into your heart!

Equipment is another big factor at the health club. One good piece of advice: pack two of everything inside your oversize gym bag. An extra water bottle sure makes one heck of a pick-up trick: "Care to quench your thirst with my big eight-ouncer?" A second Power Bar is a great way to consider a quick pit stop together over by the weight benches on your first "date." (Which makes it that much easier to rationalize sleeping with him later that same evening, since it will "officially" be your second date!) Towels are great, too. Especially if her hands are busy and you're the one who gets to dab her sweaty back. Hey, in gymspeak, that's practically getting to first base!

If all else fails, of course, and actually "working out" is too much effort for you, yet you still want to pick-up someone healthy, fit, and toned, you can always just hang out downstairs in the juice bar. Not only will you feel better downing carrot and celery juice "cocktails" instead of high balls at the local happy hour, but you also get to see what your date looks like in a leotard as well.

CAFFEINE AND POETRY: ACID REFLUX OR APHRODISIACS?

Maybe it's the fact that caffeine is cheaper than beer or wine. Maybe it's the fact that it smells better, especially when modern flavors such as cinnamon mocha frangelica and vanilla praline franceisse proliferate of late. Or maybe it's just that, if you drink enough during the shank of the evening, you're so wired by 1 or 2 a.m. that there's nothing left to do but relax with a little midnight lovin'. Either way, among the rapidly growing and culturally elite coffeehouse set, caffeine is quickly replacing oysters

"There's too much blood in my caffeine system."

— Random bumper sticker

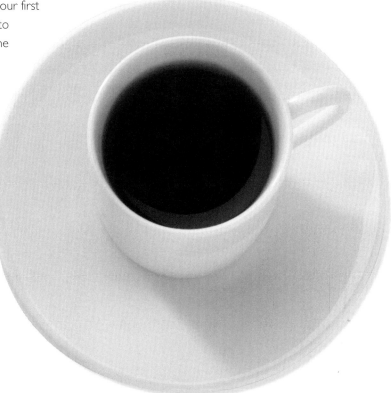

TOP-5 REASONS COFFEE IS LESS POPULAR THAN BOOZE

5 — Stained teeth much harder to get rid of than a beer belly.

4 — Caffeine buzz no match for beer buzz.

3 — Bottle is a much better phallic symbol than spoon.

2 — Ever seen a good *coffee* commercial during the Superbowl?

1 — Ever seen a coffee shop with those cool neon beer signs?

big B's have stepped in. Borders, Barnes & Noble, and Books-A-Million have all, at one time or another in recent years, opened their conveniently cozy cafés to the lofty-notion of "poetry readings."

And savvy singles have latched their romantic notions and dreams on the chance of meeting a future soul mate there, or at least a one-night stand that won't puke just after third base (unless they're allergic to coffee . . . or bad poetry).

Neon flyers plaster the front doors as you walk into your local mega-bookstore, right there in-between the MasterCard or Visa stickers and the "Shoplifters Will Be Prosecuted" sign: "Open mike poetry night, 7 p.m. this Wednesday. Bring your beret!"

as the ultimate aphrodisiac. (By the way, what's with this whole oyster thing anyway? They look like something hacked up by a three-pack-a-day smoker and are served in a dirty shell.)

Read the Friday pullout entertainment section in any town with a population larger than the word count of this sentence and you're likely to find several listings for a relatively modern phenomenon known as "open mikes." Yet no longer will the address be some seedy little downtown joint called "Books and Beans" or "Java Jim's." Nowadays the and begin scribbling fervently in those super-retro, faux-marbled, black and white Composition books. You know. The ones that you could pick up for a quarter back in the old days, but that now cost almost as much as a dark chocolate and almond biscotti.

Wearing black or beads, sporting Afros or shaved heads, tattoos or nipple rings or both, youngsters and oldsters alike show up ready to bear their soul to the masses, or at least the twenty or thirty likeminded souls crammed in to the closet-sized café. Some of the poetry may indeed be quite bad, a hybrid, amateurish blend of cryptic Kerouac free verse and flowery greeting card rhymes. Applause will be polite nonetheless, as the scent of Patchouli and Praline cream Amaretto roast fills the air. Well, why not? Everyone in the room knows that his/her name might get called next, by the weenie assistant manager who has suddenly become "the man," at least to a whole room full of heroic couplet hopefuls. Using poetry to lure a member of the opposite sex is not so easy as it might seem, however. Though the unsophisticated might be charmed by memorizing a rack of Hallmark greeting cards just before showing up at the door with a wilted bouquet of store-bought (or sidewalk picked) daisies, the typical coffeehouse hipster or hipstress is not so easily impressed. And while it may seem quite safe to assume that no one else in the room has ever heard of William Blake, the luster is guaranteed to go out of a prospective partner's eyes as soon as he finds out you've "lifted" his lines instead of carefully crafting your own. No matter how amateurish it may have sounded.

Of all the genres represented at most coffeehouse

Cautiously curious? Simply step around the piles of last month's bestsellers/this week's bargain books and notice the gleaming microphone sitting in the corner of the faux-parquet floor, surrounded by mass-produced chairs and the mandatory retro bean-bags.

Watch closely as the sideburned hipsters or wanna-beats and vampire chicks stroll in, take a seat,

—CHAPTER 10: WORKPLACE WOOING AND OTHER LAST RESORTS

or bookstore open mikes, two quickly rise to the cream of the cultural crop as surely as foam rests atop the delicate surface of a double tall latte. These are the pancake-faced, black-clad Goth set and the peppy ex-cheerleader or captain of the high school haiku team types in their alma mater sweatshirts, khaki safari pants, and Birkenstocks.

Care should be taken, when wooing one or the other, to direct one's poetry, or praise of another's poetry, accordingly. For instance, one might not aim to woo a former cast-member of *The Crow* or *Interview with the Vampire* with a poem entitled, "An Ode to the Colors of Puke Spied at My Last Kegger." Although, conversely, this same title might elicit flickering lighters and gasps among the Gap-clad groupies.

There are perks, of course, to being a coffeehouse open mike regular. Notoriety is one. While the regulars may no longer be seduced by your arched eyebrows and sedate reading style, they nonetheless recognize a familiar face and the round of resulting applause each time you step up to the mike may just be enough to turn the head of an attractive newbie.

Furthermore, most coffeehouses feature bottomless cups of coffee which, if not exactly free to begin with, at least give one the sublime appearance of having enough cash flow to "run a tab."

Although true poets consider themselves artistes (rhymes with "feasts") and would never be caught dead at an open mike, those brave souls who are into alternative dating or are at least looking to breed from a less culturally inclined gene pool might have better luck at the local karaoke bar. There, at least, folks are more honest, and dim bar lighting helps to create the illusion that one is really more talented (or at least more attractive) than one seems.

Despite the fact that most open mikes are held at so-called cafés bearing week-old bagels and slowly collapsing muffins, don't look to the open mike to replace "dinner and a movie" anytime soon. For one thing, open mikes are often held between 7 and 9 p.m. Such a schedule, of course, leaves plenty of time to go to dinner after work

and ends a little too late to satisfy the timing of an otherwise ordinary date. Also, it's hard to woo one's date with well-crafted lines poetic over the surround sound chorus of your combined stomach rumblings.

Be advised, however, that the open mike as a singles source is not for every Tom, Dick, or Sherry. While Shakespearean sonnets are not required and, indeed, rarely heard, a poetic nature is pretty hard to fake, and open mike regulars can be a tough crowd to please. Unlike the bar scene, for instance, where cheap cologne is disguised by a pervading pall of cigarette smoke and stale beer, bad poetry is easily laid bare under the fluorescent lights and expensive acoustics of today's mega-bookstores.

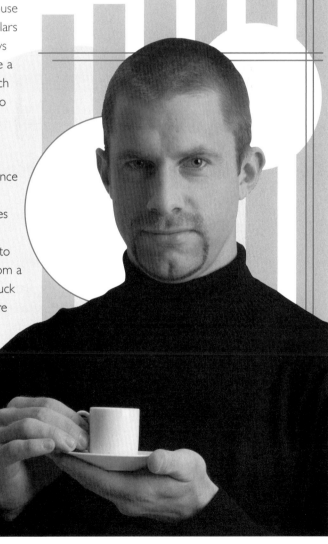

EPILOGUE

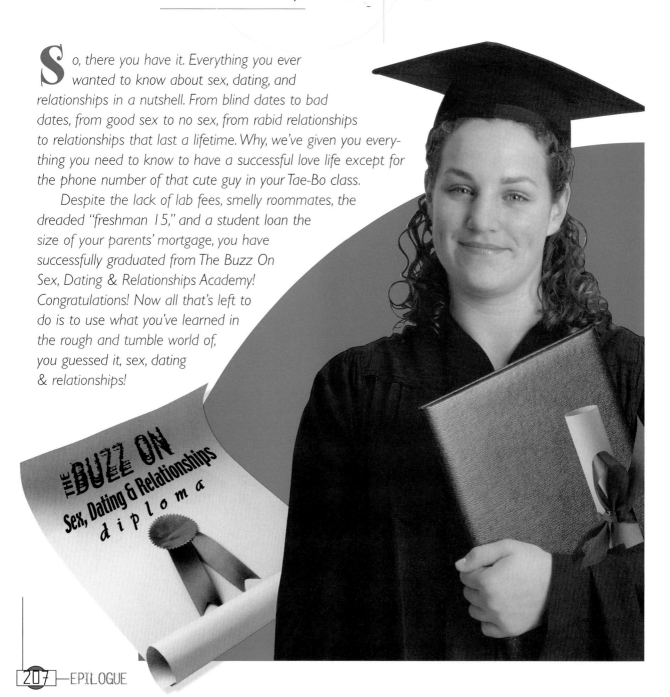

So, there you have it. Everything you ever wanted to know about sex, dating, and relationships in a nutshell. From blind dates to bad dates, from good sex to no sex, from rabid relationships to relationships that last a lifetime. Why, we've given you everything you need to know to have a successful love life except for the phone number of that cute guy in your Tae-Bo class.

Despite the lack of lab fees, smelly roommates, the dreaded "freshman 15," and a student loan the size of your parents' mortgage, you have successfully graduated from The Buzz On Sex, Dating & Relationships Academy! Congratulations! Now all that's left to do is to use what you've learned in the rough and tumble world of, you guessed it, sex, dating & relationships!

AFTER (WORD) THE LOVIN'

Through it all, we've tried to help you learn more about love, more about sex, but mostly, learn more about yourself. What type of a date are you interested in? What kind of relationship do you want? Who are you and who do you want to be with? How much are you willing to put up with so you don't have to be alone? Do you really even mind being alone in the first place?

Sure, it's been fun. But we hope you learned a little something along the way. Maybe you picked up a tip on spicing up your love life that actually worked. Perhaps you got wise to the wacky world of online personal ads. Or maybe you even worked up the nerve to ask that hot little number in your car pool out? Either way, you're guaranteed to have the latest buzz on not just sex, not just dating, and not just relationships—but all three!

Naturally, your education doesn't end here. (That's why it's called a reference guide. Otherwise, it would have been called a brain transplant!) Use the helpful information provided here on your next date, or use it to help you get that next date. Flirt better, listen more, and, for heaven's sake, if you're going to indulge in trashy, tasteless, titillating one-night stands, don't forget to hide the coffeemaker before he wakes up the next morning! (You wouldn't want him sticking around all day, now would you?)

And, now that you're armed with the lethal weapons you'll need to win the battle of the sexes, it's only a matter of time before the love of your life appears in your sights. Will you know what to do? Sure you will. (Now, anyway.) And who knows? By the time you're married and settled down, with the kids in college and nothing else to do but suffer through a particularly bad case of empty nest syndrome, there might even be a *Buzz On Sex, Dating & Relationships #2: The Golden Years!*

Hey, who said sex, dating, and relationships are only for the young folks?

TOP-5 REASONS YOU'LL BE SAD WHEN THIS BOOK IS OVER

5.) "Now where will I use my *Playgirl* bookmark?"

4.) "I dunno, that Max guy was kinda cute!"

3.) "Hey, where's my free blow-up doll?"

2.) Now you have to take that thirty page quiz your girlfriend's prepared for you.

1.) No more **Top-5** lists! (Come on, we know you love 'em.)

Jaws, 4, 95
Jerry Maguire, 110
Jingle Cats, 29
Joan of Arc, 7
Johnson, Howard, 93
Johnson's, Howard, 93
Jungle Jim's, 75

K

Kama Sutra, 27, 125
Keaton, Diane, 10
Kennedy, Jamie, 93
Kent, Clark, 40
Kermit (the frog), 9
Kidman, Nicole, 97
Kill, Baby, Kill!, 3
Kilmer, Val, 102
King, Stephen, 35-36
kissing
as a lost art, 15
as a surprise, 18
at ballgames, 17
at red lights, 18
at weddings, 18
during racquetball, 18
timing of, 16
under the mistletoe, 17
variety in, 16
Korn, 182

L

ladies night (*see* also bars)
  he said, 85-87
  she said, 83-85
Lady & the Tramp, 101
Landon, Michael, 9
lang, k. d., 131
Last Horror Film, The, 3
Las Vegas, 171
Laundromats

Laundromats (continued)
  as places to meet people, 197-199
  pick-up lines, 199
Leave It to Beaver, 158
Le Langage des Fleurs, 20
Lee, Tommy, 106
Lee, Jason, 102
Leigh, Vivien, 10
Leno, Jay, 77
Let's Scare Jessica to Death, 3
Levenson, Sam 34
Life is Beautiful, 109
Lifetime, Television for Women, 105
Lion King, The, 95
Longest Yard, The, 101
Louganis, Greg, 131
Lovett, Lyle, 99
Lumiére, Louis, 92

M

MacLaine, Shirley, 10
Madonna, 10
make-out albums (list), 17
making love (survey), 186
Mallrats, 102
Manilow, Barry, 29
Manson, Marilyn, 11
marriage (*see* also wedding
  reception)
  as a legal agreement, 156
  benefits (list), 158
  Elizabeth Taylor, 9-10
  history of, 156-158
  survey, 157
  types of (list), 156
  wedding ceremony, 169-170
Marx, Groucho, 46, 146
Mary Tyler Moore, 145
McBeal, Ally, 185, 187
McDonald's, 58, 94
Medieval (pick-up lines), 6

X

Y

Z